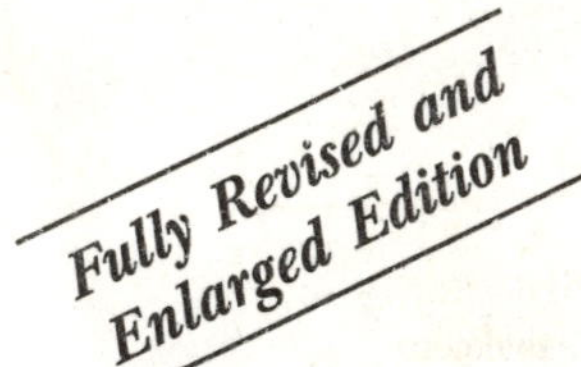

Slim & Smart Body

A fitness programme for men & women

Barun Roy

PUSTAK MAHAL®

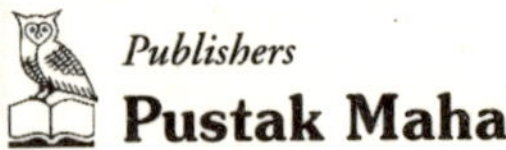

Publishers
Pustak Mahal®

J-3/16 , Daryaganj, New Delhi-110002
☎ 23276539, 23272783, 23272784 • *Fax:* 011-23260518
E-mail: info@pustakmahal.com • *Website:* www.pustakmahal.com

Sales Centre

- 10-B, Netaji Subhash Marg, Daryaganj, New Delhi-110002
  ☎ 23268292, 23268293, 23279900 • *Fax:* 011-23280567
  E-mail: rapidexdelhi@indiatimes.com
- 6686, Khari Baoli, Delhi-110006
  ☎ 23944314, 23911979

Branches

Bengaluru: ☎ 080-22234025 • *Telefax:* 080-22240209
E-mail: pustak@airtelmail.in • pustak@sancharnet.in
Mumbai: ☎ 022-22010941, 022-22053387
E-mail: rapidex@bom5.vsnl.net.in
Patna: ☎ 0612-3294193 • *Telefax:* 0612-2302719
E-mail: rapidexptn@rediffmail.com
Hyderabad: *Telefax:* 040-24737290
E-mail: pustakmahalhyd@yahoo.co.in

ISBN 978-81-223-0782-5

Edition: 2012

Printed at : Param Offsetters, Okhla, New Delhi-110020

Dedicated to the memory of

Sailesh Pradhan (1977-2001)

the best friend I ever had....

Acknowledgement

This book and my physical well-being are the result of a comment my dear friend Debashis Sengupta once made when I was 20 kg overweight and a chain-smoker. He met me in the market, looked at me and blurted out, "What's wrong with you? You look like an elephant!" Although I received many comments like that, Debashis' words sank home because he himself was 25 kg overweight! In many ways, this book should be dedicated to him.

My younger brother, Baijnath Roy, had always been the main hand behind this book, while I wrote and researched for the same in Kolkata. It was indeed an unconscious slip of mind on a gigantic scale that I simply forgot to even mention his name in the first edition. This second edition, hence, I would like to dedicate in part to him for having been with me in Kolkata through the entire period when the first edition of this book was conceived.

There has been much that has also changed in my life during the last few years. I traveled through almost half of the globe, lost hearing on my right ear in an explosion and came close to being drafted in the Georgian Army. But the best of all, I finally gathered strength and courage to say 'Yes' to marriage and settle down. Of course, the crucial step has not yet been taken but I have faith that it won't be much of a problem. As a mark of love and respect to my future muse, Samjhana Subba, thence, who takes keen interest in my work, I thank her and hope that she inspires me to come up with more such literary works.

I am also grateful to my numerous friends and, most importantly, to the readers who wrote back to me by post and email, embracing at the same time all that the book embodied. It is their acceptance which made the first edition of Slim and Smart Body a bestseller. I thank them with all my heart.

Contents

Preface

Most of the people who know me well will wonder why a man, who was once a chain-smoker and 20 kg overweight, chose to write a book on fitness. Here is the answer: I went through what most of you are going today. I used to look at fit people and say, "*Man, how in God's name can I be something like that?*" I tried numerous remedies. Pills, more pills. I joined numerous gyms, worked out like anything and ended with a sore back and a bad mood. However, I realized that the problem was actually inside me. There was no need for expensive gyms, pills, and so on. It just required simple workouts. But I must make one thing clear here. I am not going to suggest any magic fitness programme. You can jog, you can hop, or you can dance if you wish . Anything that involves moving limbs and spending energy is a workout for me. In addition, done properly and regularly, these exercises work wonders for us. Through this book, I just want to share something that has changed my life.

Everyone wants to be fit. We envy fitness. To have clean muscular lines, to be strong, to be flexible and graceful – the visible signs of well-being as well as of confidence and presence – are traits desired by everyone. Have you ever seen a fat gymnast or a pot-bellied model? Have you noticed how concerned and alive diet-conscious athletes are at parties?

Some people make weak excuses about food, fitness and exercise; but they are actually fat, lazy and jealous of those who are fit. They almost feel threatened while in the company of fit people.

In addition, another strange thing is that fitness is available to everyone who can walk and even to those who cannot. It is one of the few things life offers that no one can say is not essential.

This book is designed to make fitness accessible to you while acquaiting you with the basic idea of fitness. However, this is just a guide. I have deliberately left a lot for you to explore and discover yourself. The reason I have done this is because there is no greater adventure than exploring the realm of possibilities yourself. I, for one, am sure that you will surprise yourself.

So welcome to a new world, a world where you will challenge yourself, where you will be proud of yourself and where you will be fit.

Spring 2004 **–Barun Roy**
Clarke Road, Darjeeling

Some things I must express....

Since its first edition, Slim and Smart Body was widely accepted by readers. Everything set in motion in the book also seems to have, like a huge jigsaw puzzle, been solved and demystified. A letter from Jodhpur, from a young man who was 30 kg overweight telling me that he lost 10 kg or a similar email from a Mumbai homemaker telling me that she lost 6 kg and is today not just an active participant in all social activities but one who for the first time in her life leads others, are indeed remarkable success stories. The list of such appreciations and confirmation of the ideas endorsed by the book is simply unending.

However, this does not go on to say that the book in itself or my humble self should indulge in self boasting for I am simply not the one who made it happen. Let's be frank, any book in itself is simply words, just words. It is the readers, who bring life to the book by practicing it, making it thus, really valuable. Slim and Smart Body is just such a book which the readers, through their active participation made a bestseller and even better than that, successful in terms of its practicality and worth in real life and for real people.

When I set out to update and essentially rewrite this book for the third edition, I did not feel the need to change either the format or even rewrite most of the chapters. They were already complete and rewriting the same would have only lead to confusion, hence, I thought it well to instead include a new section at the end of the book which contained discussions of some of the things that I had not already indulged in. This involves simple yet important things. Things like sleep. For how often do we take our sleep to be important? With the fast pace of life that we are accustomed with and the steep career graph that we chase; sleep does not seem to be at the top of our mind. Similarly, our food habits, how and what we should eat. How much we should drink? All these questions and more, indeed have been answered.

Similarly, there were certain mails which asked me to discuss some fitness regimen for elderly people. There were even some who have been physically challenged, yet still wanted to have a 'slim and smart' body. It was essential that I include some chapters for them. 'Walking our way to a healthy life', has hence, been included to make people aware of the benefits of such simple thing as walking, which is perhaps the best of all exercises.

I was also made aware of a rather unique problem by one Mr. Inder from Bhopal, who sent me an email, asking me to specify some exercises for him. His problem a rather persistent one originated due to his work, which essentially consisted of working on the computer for almost ten hours. 'Computers could be a health hazard – How do you avoid this' is a chapter solely intended towards, millions of computer professionals like Inder all over the nation.

Frequently Asked Questions (FAQ) Section has been updated and upgraded.

This edition also includes improved format, with better diagrams, pictures, illustrations and data sheets. There are sample chart and sheets you can now use to trace and maintain your health. Glossary has been updated and new terms and concepts explained.

Above all, this edition should be well accepted by the readers as the previous editions.

So welcome again to a new world, a world where you will challenge yourself, where you will be proud of yourself and where you will be fit.

–Barun Roy

What is Fitness?

At the very outset it is really important to know what we mean when we talk about fitness. Of course, there are many definitions of fitness. However, the definition on which most of the experts agree is as follows:

Fitness: It is the Ability of Your Body to Cope with Stress

This includes mental and physical stress. If you decide to perform a difficult task, it is better if you know in advance how much stress your body can bear. Armed with this knowledge and understanding of your own body and its fitness level, you can exert yourself freely with much more ease. But, if you do it without proper understanding, the same task may prove quite risky and you may even harm yourself.

For example, you may decide to run 10 km or to do a bench press of 420 pounds[1]. Of course, you are not trained sufficiently and as a consequence, two things might happen: you will make it and pay for it in post-exercise pain, agony and despair, or you just won't make it and still despair. The conclusion is that you didn't have the fitness level necessary to cope with the level of stress of a 10 km run or 420 kg bench press placed upon you.

However, in any case, it is not easy to run 10 km at a stretch or lift 420 kg. Why? Because, it needs a very high

[1] 2.2pounds = 1kg

fitness level, which normally we don't have[2]. But, for that matter, do we possess the fitness level to cope with everyday life?

a. Flexibility Test

A measuring tape or 36 inch ruler is required for this test. This test should be done after a short warm-up for the lower back and hamstring muscles. The individual should be seated with shoes removed and with legs outstretched and feet 10 inches apart. Insure that legs are flat on the floor and not bent. The measuring tape is positioned with the 15-inch mark at the heels and the zero mark towards the body. With the hands crossed and fingers even, the individual under test reaches forward and holds momentarily while measurement is taken. Take three trials and record the highest reading. Consult the table below.

MEN	**20's**	**30's**	**40's**	**50's**	**60's**
Excellent	22+	21+	20+	19+	18+
Good	16 - 21	15 - 20	14 - 19	13 - 18	12 - 17
Average	13 - 15	12 - 14	11 - 13	10 - 12	9 - 11
Below Avg	below 13	below 12	below 11	below 10	below 9

WOMEN	**20's**	**30's**	**40's**	**50's**	**60's**
Excellent	19+	18+	17+	16+	15+
Good	13 - 18	12 - 17	11 - 16	10 - 15	9 - 14
Average	10 - 12	9 - 11	8 - 10	7 - 9	6 - 8
Below Avg	below 10	below 9	below 8	below 7	below 6

[2] It could be an interesting experience testing one's fitness level before planning a training regimen. The International Fitness Association (IFA) has recommended the following fitness tests:

b. Pushup Test

The individual to be tested should lie on the floor in the prone position with the hands pointed forward and immediately under the shoulders. Start with the chin touching the floor then push up by straightening the arms. Instruct the individual to maintain body alignment as they push up.

For males, the legs should be extended out and positioned together using the feet as pivots. For females, the upper leg should be straight out using the knees as pivots. There is no time limit for this test. Instruct the individual to complete as many pushups as they can. Discontinue the test when the individual begins to exhibit straining. Consult the table below.

MEN	teens	20's	30's	40's	50's	60's
Excellent	45+	39+	33+	27+	24+	23+
Good	31 - 41	26 - 35	22 - 29	18 - 25	15 - 22	14 - 20
Average	26 - 29	22 - 25	18 - 21	15 - 17	12 - 14	10 - 13
Below Avg	14 - 24	12 - 21	9 - 17	7 - 14	5 - 11	3 - 9
Poor	below 14	below 12	below 9	below 7	below 5	below 3

WOMEN	teens	20's	30's	40's	50's	60's
Excellent	31+	30+	29+	24+	20+	18+
Good	21 - 28	19 - 26	18 - 26	15 - 22	12 - 18	11 – 16
Average	17 - 20	16 - 18	14 - 17	12 - 14	10 - 12	8 - 10
Below Avg	9 - 16	8 - 15	5 - 13	4 - 11	3 - 9	2 - 7
Poor	below 9	below 8	below 5	below 4	below 3	below 2

With increased leisure time today and the availability of many new activities to all of us, increase in fitness levels can widen our horizons. Besides, this would strengthen our body and develop its disease resistance capacity. A proper fitness level also reduces the risks of heart disease and other such fatal attacks. And above all, we can enjoy the peace of mind and a great feeling of well being with a sound body.

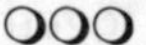

First Step: Mind Holds the Key

Other books might suggest specific gears you would need for your workouts or the type of workouts you should do. Not me. Most of the fitness programmes fail because they miss the first most important step. This is called mental preparation.

One morning you decide to go for exercise. You wear your runners and your tracksuit and come out in the fresh air for jogging. By the time you have jogged for 10 minutes, you are already very tired. You curse yourself. The pain is unbearable and you feel you were happy without this exercise. Prove that I am wrong. Tell me that it hasn't happened with you.

Most people go to gyms for the first time and leave it saying, "*That's it, never again in my life.*" And they are not wrong. We human beings are basically restless and lack patience. We want to look like Brad Pitt or Arnie in just one week. If this was not so, why would wonder pills and drugs sell like hot cakes all over the world?

You should not start your exercise after you wake up one day with a '*let's-be-fit*' mood. You should first prepare your mind and convince yourself that this is something you really need. You should stand before the mirror and say, "*I am cute but I have a great capability to be cuter. My arms are thinner and my body needs to be more muscular.*" That's it! That's your first workout. You should make yourself feel bad about your own situation. If you are fat and that's how you like it, then let me tell you … you are fine the way you are. However, if you want to change your situation, if you are tired of being called a fatty or skinny, or if a person you love ignores you, then it's time you prove what you really are.

Anyone can be fit. It does not really matter what you do. It can be bodybuilding, gymnastics, aerobics or just plain jogging. Remember, the first battle to be fought is right in your mind. You will first have to convince yourself that you are tired of being unfit. Then you are ready for workouts.

Another very important thing that occurs at this stage is the feeling of 'I *can't do it*'. I still remember the first time I wore my running shoes and went for jogging in Chowrasta, Darjeeling. After just 10 minutes, I was panting and coughing. Years of chain-smoking had done the damage. However, since I was mentally prepared, I kept my calm, smiled and started walking. It is true that I was not able to jog a long distance, but I enjoyed whatever distance I had jogged. The idea here is to feel good, to feel fit. You have to gear up your mind for that. You will have to say, "*I jogged for five minutes yesterday, today it was six minutes.*" For you, it is a great achievement. Don't ever compare with other people. They might be jogging on their head and you might be struggling with your legs, but that's alright.

❍❍❍

How to Start?

One really good thing about fitness training is the fact that you don't need to rush out and purchase expensive equipment. Most of the gear that you'll need, you probably already have. It should be comfortable. Look good and feel good–is the simple mantra for the beginners.

However, there are a few sensible precautions one should take before entering into any fitness programme straight from a sedentary lifestyle.

It is essential that the first thing you do is to have a thorough medical examination and tell your doctor what you intend to do. Most doctors fully support daily exercise and understand the value of preventative measures, one of the things fitness training is all about. However, if you are in your early twenties (or under) and play outdoor games and have no previous medical problems, this precaution is unnecessary. But the following people should have a thorough medical check-up before undertaking any fitness programme:

- Inactive people over the age of 25
- People who are chain-smokers
- People who are alcoholics
- People who are overweight by more than 7 kg
- People with any heart or lung associated illness
- Women who are pregnant

Embarking on a fitness programme requires a green signal from the doctor for these people. Once you have it and have already 'prepared' your mind, here's what I recommend you wear:

- Shorts with an elastic waistband or leotards. Track pants when it is cold.
- T-shirt.
- Sports socks – the cotton, padded ones preferably.
- Runners.
- Headbands–they look good and help absorb the sweat that troubles your eyes as it runs down your forehead.
- Tracksuit or windcheater to keep on during your warm-ups in winter and to put on again after your workout so that you do not get a chill after you cool down.

Quality of Runners

Which runners suit you the best for fitness training?

There is a huge range of runners to choose from and most people decide which pair they'll buy following the advice of the sales staff in the shoe or sports store. So how should you decide about a good training shoe for your particular fitness programme? Magazines about fitness conduct surveys on various brands by comparing designs and functions and provide a categorical list of their various features. These magazines often prove very helpful and informative. You can consult these magazines.

The efficiency and quality of a training shoe is not always geared to the price–some reasonably priced shoes are just as good as, and often a lot better than, the very expensive models.

Now, you have everything you need to get started. Remember, today is the beginning of the rest of your life.

OOO

What is Aerobics?

Try asking a friend what aerobics means and you'll probably get answers like 'exercising to music' or 'dancing exercise'. It is sad to know how many well-intentioned people miss the real benefits of aerobics. Though they try hard, they fail to achieve the result because of lack of understanding of what they are doing or due to want of proper guidance. Often, a bit of music and a few routines are all they get. And that is certainly not what aerobics is all about.

The word 'aerobics' came into everyday use because of the popularity of exercise-to-music classes, but it actually means something completely different. It's a word that is quite hard to explain clearly and simply until we know something about a science called **Physiology**.

Physiology is an interesting subject. With tremendous development in the field of science and technology, and especially in biology and medical science, we have been able to know our body much better. Our understanding about what actually makes our body tick has widened enormously. However, when the human machine is studied under conditions of physical training, this subject becomes quite fascinating. I hope you'll persevere with the bio-chemistry coming up. Even if you find it irrelevant at first, I know the conclusion will be of interest.

If you look up the meaning of the word 'aerobic' in a dictionary, it is given as 'occurring in the presence of oxygen', which is not of much help. I hope to make clear what takes place in the presence of oxygen inside our body and why aerobic fitness is such a wonderful quality to possess.

Oxygen is a gas. The air we breathe is made up of different gases comprising mainly nitrogen and oxygen. Air is 79 per cent nitrogen. We breathe it in and out of our lungs daily but we never use any of it. Actually we breathe 79 per cent nitrogen in and 79 per cent out again.

However, air also contains 21 per cent oxygen. We breathe 21 per cent oxygen in but we exhale less. Our bodies use oxygen to burn the digested food material. The amount of oxygen we consume depends on what we're doing. If a person is sleeping or sitting, he wouldn't consume much, but if he is running or taking part in some form of endurance (long-term) exercise, his body would consume a lot more.

Another gas in the air is carbon dioxide. There is very little carbon dioxide in the air we breathe in but, because this is the gas human beings produce as a waste material, there is quite a lot of carbon dioxide in the air we breathe out. This process of absorption of oxygen and emission of carbon dioxide is known as respiration.

What happens to the oxygen once it has been absorbed into the bloodstream? The answer is that this oxygen is consumed to enable you to produce energy.

What exactly is 'energy'? Let's stop here and look at some forms of energy present on Earth: nuclear, electrical, solar, chemical, mechanical and heat energy. In all cases, energy is the 'capacity to do work'.

All forms of energy can be converted from one form to another. For example, chemical energy, like food and oxygen, can be changed into mechanical energy, such as human movement.

It is this energy transformation (chemical energy into mechanical energy) which takes place in the presence of oxygen. The process is called aerobic metabolism.

Food consists of fats, carbohydrates and proteins. Our bodies have the ability to break down foods and either store them as fat deposits or use them to produce energy. When we use food for energy we break the food down into glucose. Glucose is stored in the liver, fat cells and other storage areas of the body. Your blood can retrieve glucose and make it ready for muscle cells to 'use' as a source of energy. The blood carries this glucose or sugar around to the millions of cells in the body, where the 'energy process' takes place.

So it is true to say that aerobic metabolism takes place inside each cell. Obviously, the cells referred to are mainly muscle cells.

There are millions of cells in our body, each one performing its specific jobs to maintain life. It is possible to study these cells under a microscope and, thus, scientists have discovered the mechanics of cellular activity. Not everything is known about cellular activity, but the mechanism for aerobic energy production has been known since 1953. But still, even today, some of the secrets of aerobic metabolism remain unknown. Here, we are simply concerned with the conversion of chemical energy (food) into mechanical energy (muscular movement).

The energy released during the breakdown of the food one eats is not directly used for human movement. There is a vital in-between step we must look at. The energy released during the breakdown of food is used to form another chemical known as **adenosine tri-phosphate** (ATP). This chemical is stored in all muscle cells, and only by the breakdown of ATP can energy be released for the cell to perform its work, that is, muscular contractions.

Some scientists have called ATP the 'energy currency of the body'. Now that we know the immediate source of energy, which enables a muscle to contract, we have to ask how it is supplied.

There are three ways: the ATP-PC system, glycolysis or lactic acid system, and aerobic metabolism.

The subject we are discussing here is known as **bioenergetics**, one of the most fascinating areas of science.

The ATP-PC System

ATP is present in all muscle cells. Another chemical, **phosphocreatine** (PC) is also present in all muscle cells. There is always more PC stored in muscle cells than ATP, because PC is used to make ATP. When the muscle needs ATP (for muscular contraction) PC is 'broken down', releasing energy and ATP is formed. When the ATP is broken down, energy is released. Part of the energy is used to allow the muscle to contract and some of the energy is used to put the PC back together again. So, the only way PC can be re-formed is from the energy released due to the breakdown of ATP when work is done. Also, ATP can be re-formed due to the breakdown of PC.

Understanding of ATP-PC system is important if you choose to 'train' in your gym. Because you are interested in powerful, quick-start sports like the shotput, short sprints etc., your training programme should include specific exercises designed to develop this energy system–quick, short bursts of very intense activity on your legs if you are a sprinter or high jumper, for example. This system does not involve a series of chemical reactions nor does it require oxygen; therefore, it is the fastest available source of ATP production for muscular contraction. Because the ATP-PC system requires no oxygen, it is described as an 'anaerobic' source of energy. It is also limited: it cannot produce very much ATP and therefore, cannot provide the muscle with the ability to complete work over extended periods. Unlike the other two energy suppliers, it is not a metabolic pathway.

The Lactic Acid System (Glycolysis)

This energy system was discovered in the 1930s by two German scientists. It is often called **glycolysis** which means 'sugar dissolved'. It takes place inside the muscle cell and is anaerobic (i.e. it does not require oxygen). This energy system involves the partial breakdown of food. The only food this system can use is carbohydrate, broken down into glucose. The glucose is stored in the liver and in muscle, and in its 'stored state' is called **glycogen**. This energy system uses glucose as 'food fuel' purely for the production of ATP. The glucose is present inside the muscle cell and produces the ATP the muscle needs to contract. What happens to the glucose? Through a complicated series of chemical reactions, the glucose is broken down, step by step, until it ends up as lactic acid. During the step-by-step breakdown, ATP is produced and supplied to the muscle to do work. However, like the ATP-PC system, not much ATP is produced – for every molecule of glucose that undergoes glycolysis, only two molecules of ATP are supplied to the muscle. Nevertheless, like the ATP-PC energy system, the lactic acid system is very important to us, because it supplies a very quick supply of ATP to the muscle for activities which depend on maximum effort for two or three minutes like sprints, relays, long jump, which all depend upon energy (ATP) supplied from the ATP-PC and lactic acid systems.

Again, when you work out at your gym, the fitness-training programme you select should be geared to the kind of activities you pursue in everyday life. To develop these anaerobic energy systems by completing training programmes with short-burst/maximum effort content when you are a marathon runner, for example, would be senseless. That kind of programme is tailored for the sprinter etc. Rather, the marathon/distance endurance athlete would have to concentrate upon the third and last of these energy systems: aerobic metabolism.

The Oxygen System–Aerobic Metabolism

Here we are going to find out what aerobics really is. If we go back to the lactic acid system, I mentioned the glucose molecule being broken down through a series of very complicated chemical reactions until it ends up as lactic acid. In the oxygen system, if oxygen is in abundant supply, all the glucose molecules will not end up as lactic acid. The glucose reaction will end up one chemical reaction short, in the form of pyruvate.

So, if oxygen is present, the glucose molecule breakdown process (glycolysis) is 'sidetracked' when it has been broken down as far as pyruvate, and this pyruvate then enters into the oxygen system – or aerobic metabolism.

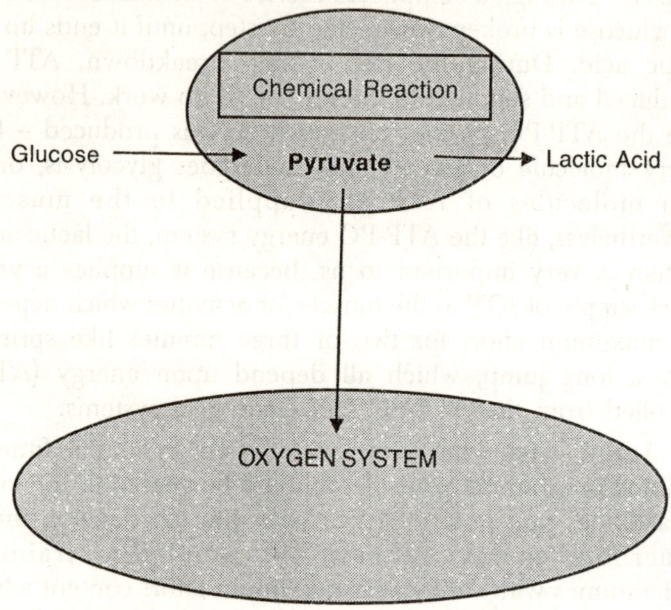

How are Two Energy Systems Linked?

This discovery was made in 1953 by Hans Kreb (later Sir Hans). Kreb was awarded a Nobel Prize for this discovery and the oxygen system was named after him – the Kreb's Cycle. Kreb also discovered that the oxygen system could utilize fats (fatty acids) and proteins (amino acids) as well as glucose as fuel to create ATP. Present in the cell are glucose, fats and proteins. The ATP-PC and Lactic Acid systems are limited because their only food fuel is glycogen/glucose – not so aerobic metabolism.

The process of the lactic acid system takes place inside the cell and, as a consequence, pyruvate is present inside it too. So are the fatty acids and amino acids. Similar to the way glucose is converted into pyruvate, fatty acids and amino acids are converted into acetoacetic acid. Inside the cell a small organelle (or structure) called a mitochondrion exists which is called the 'power house' of the cell. And inside the mitochondria is where the third energy system takes place.

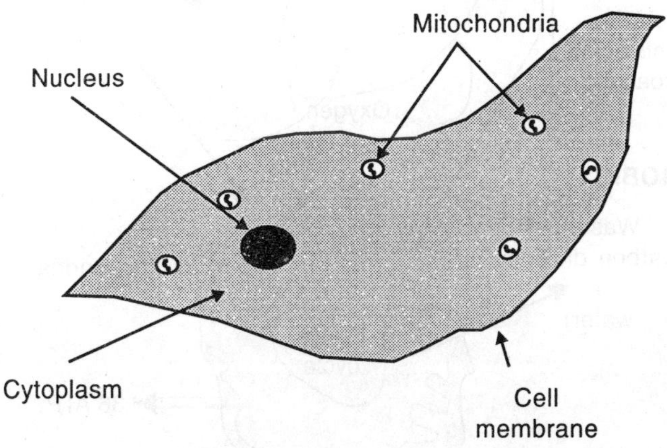

Diagram of Muscle Cell

Kreb studied the cell and noticed that the pyruvate along with the acetoacetic acid, both present in the cell, were together being formed into another chemical known as acetyl co-enzyme A, and this new substance was being funneled off into these mitochondria. He noticed that oxygen was also being funneled off into the mitochondria and when this phenomenon took place 36 molecules of ATP were produced for every molecule of fuel - enough ATP to produce 18 times the energy produced by the lactic acid system. This was his discovery - the Kreb's Cycle.

Let's re cap with the diagram below.

ATP Energy Results of Two Energy Systems

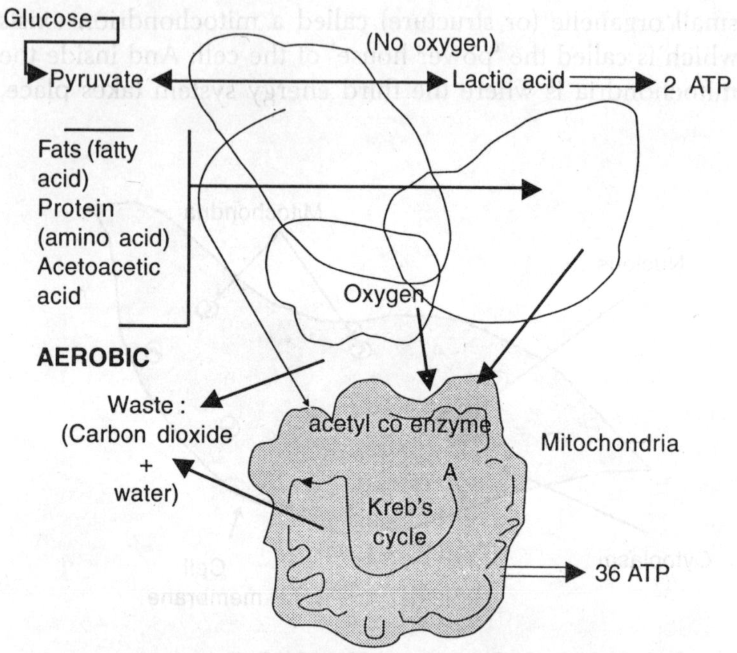

As you can see the end products of the oxygen system (Kreb's Cycle) are carbon dioxide and water. It is simple now to understand why we breathe oxygen in and carbon dioxide out.

From this knowledge has stemmed a huge amount of scientific application in the training of athletes. Coaches and trainers have obviously concentrated their efforts on providing their athletes with training programmes which emphasize the development of their energy systems as much as the development of techniques and strategies.

The importance of the science of bioenergetics has been reflected in the continued ability of men and women in breaking world records in almost every physical individual sporting and athletic event.

But how do you know which energy system your body is using and how long does each one last? Of course, it's going to depend on what activity you're involved with. So let's start with your body the way it is now: reading this book.

You are presently at rest, and believe it or not, you are producing your energy aerobically. Why is this so? Your heart-lung system is just ticking over nice and slowly while you are at rest (heart rate around 72 beats per minute). Because you are resting, your blood (which carries oxygen) is capable of carrying enough oxygen to each cell and, therefore, satisfying the energy requirements of 'the resting state'.

What about the two ATP molecules from the lactic acid system? Well, because oxygen is present, and there is no change in the lactic acid levels contained in your blood at rest (about 10 mg/100 ml of blood), the two ATP molecules are included with the aerobic contribution of ATP. (Seems like we're cheating here a bit, but not until blood lactic acid levels rise do we really consider anaerobic energy systems to be primary contributors to energy supply.)

'Rest' has been discussed, but what about energy supply under conditions of exercise? Well, this section of the chapter is absolutely crucial when you consider any form of physical training, because it will depend on the intensity and duration of your training bouts as to which energy system you are actually improving.

This has proved a constant source of amazement to me, as I have seen aerobic classes with high-intensity running and jumping sections last only two or three minutes, which obviously is not 'aerobic' but is 'anaerobic', because as soon as this 'burst' is over, they move into low key, slow pace movements and, therefore, defeat the whole purpose of the class. I hope you haven't been attending such classes, because if you have, you have been wasting your time and money, actually speaking.

To continue my discussion, here I'll divide all exercises into two categories:

1. Exercises performed for a short time and at high intensity.
2. Exercises performed for longer periods and at medium intensity.

Exercise for a Short Time at High Intensity

Events described here include 100-metre races, relays, push-ups, sit-ups, sprints up to 800 metres and other activities, where activity can be maintained for 2 to 3 minutes. The major food-fuel is glucose. The predominant energy supply is anaerobic.

It is a mistake, however, to assume that the aerobic system is not working. It is working, but not very much. We say we are working 'anaerobically' when the aerobic system cannot supply ATP alone, and it needs to be supplemented with ATP provided by the ATP-PC and lactic acid systems. When we do exercises in this category, you might ask why the aerobic system cannot provide adequate ATP straightaway. One reason is that each of us can only 'consume' a certain 'amount' of oxygen and if you go running in full blast for 100 metres, you would have to be able to consume about 15 times the maximum amount of oxygen anyone can consume to do it on the oxygen system alone. Another reason for having implemented the ATP-PC system and the lactic acid system is that the oxygen system needs 2 or 3 minutes to get itself going, i.e. increases in heart rate, breathing etc.

To conclude this section on exercise performed for a short time at high intensity, discussion of lactic acid is essential. If you look back to the lactic acid system (glycolysis) of ATP production, you can see that in the absence of oxygen, the end product of glycolysis is, in fact, lactic acid.

As the glucose is used for fuel in the lactic acid system, so also lactic acid accumulates in the muscles and in the blood. (Remember, this is in the absence of oxygen!) With very high levels of lactic acid in the blood and inside the muscles, the muscles cannot contract any more, and that's why you feel fatigued or tired after an intense 3-minute burst of exercise. The exercise must stop or you must have a break! This accumulation of lactic acid is known as 'oxygen debt', and when this state is reached, the athlete has to wait until more oxygen has been consumed so that the lactic acid levels are reduced and exercise can continue. This lactic acid buildup is depleted by the presence of oxygen converting the lactic acid back to pyruvate and then this pyruvate moving through into the oxygen system (Kreb's Cycle).

This is interesting because really top athletes have the ability to withstand enormous amounts of lactic acid levels in their muscles and blood before they slow down or stop, and because they can tolerate such high levels, they just keep going when the others have succumbed to lactic acid build-up effects.

Next time when you go to gym and complete a work-out, especially if it's an 'aerobic' class, if you do a short 'run-jump', then a stretch, then a jog, then some tummy work, then another jog – in fact, if the programme consists of a disjointed array of short bursts on various muscle groups, then you know you are not working out aerobically at all.

Exercise for Longer Periods at Medium Intensity

The kinds of exercises here are activities which take longer than 5 to 10 minutes at a minimum to complete. Running and swimming long distances and sustained cycling are good examples. The best example in this category is the marathon runner, as this event is one where the athlete is running for over two and a half hours over a distance of 42 km or 26 miles – a real fun day out, eh?

In these types of exercises, the major source of ATP is provided by the oxygen system – true aerobic metabolism. The other two energy systems are employed right at the beginning for 2 or 3 minutes but once the oxygen consumed reaches its new level and the muscle cells start to receive supplies of oxygen, no lactic acid build-up will occur and therefore, exercise can continue.

Through correct training, an efficient heart-lung system can develop and oxygen can be quickly and efficiently carried to the cells where the oxygen system can produce abundant supplies of ATP. Energy supplies can be increased and achievements in physical endurance events can be accomplished. After these prolonged 'endurance' training programmes, athletes still feel tired, but not because they have built up lactic acid; they haven't, because they were working aerobically. So why do they feel so fatigued after each workout?

There are several reasons, but primarily because they have depleted sugar stores in their muscles and their liver. Another reason is that they have lost water – dehydration – and they should replenish this with drinks after the event. No, not booze! Water is what you should take. There is a modern technique used to overcome this shortage of sugar in muscles and liver after a very long endurance event, say over 2 hours in duration, and even though you may never complete such a huge physical challenge, it may interest you to read this example of science and human movement.

It is known as **super saturation** or **carbo-hydrate loading** and it involves saturating your muscles and liver with sugar. You might have heard about marathon runners eating carbohydrate rich food. It's to do with that kind of thing. The problem here is most people don't realize it, but that bowl of food won't help much unless the correct procedure of super saturation is followed for a period of six or seven days.

Please remember, before you attempt physical endurance activity of this calibre, a sensible, specific training programme must be adhered to for a period of three to six months before the event.

The level of glycogen/glucose contained in a muscle remains at a fairly steady level during day-to-day life, but as mentioned, extensive endurance exercise causes this level to fall, leaving muscles depleted.

How then do athletes super saturate or load carbohydrate? Six to seven days before an important event the athlete will exhaust the muscles (used in that event) of stored glycogen (this requires approximately 120 to 160 minutes of activity at medium intensity). And then, for Days Six, Five and Four before the important event, the athlete follows a diet consisting of fat and protein. He or she will eat foods rich in protein and fat. Also, on Days Six, Five and Four, endurance activity (specific to the event) is maintained. This gets really hard: you're hanging out for a cake by the time Day Four arrives! OK, you make it to the third day before

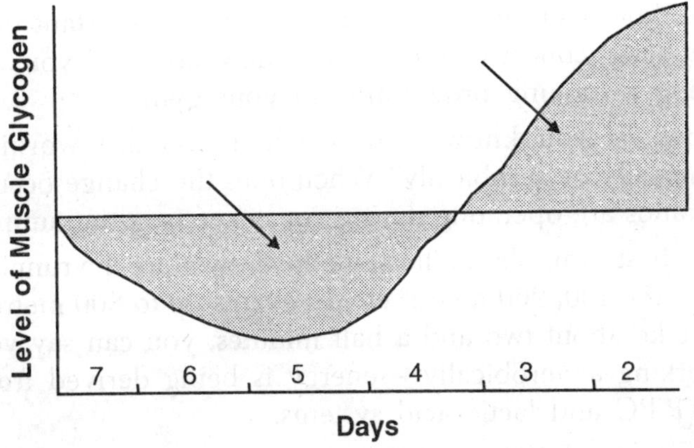

the event and you get the chance to pig out on all those high carbohydrate foods, therefore, maintaining a high-energy carbohydrate diet for the last three days. Foods in this category are cakes, chocolate, milkshakes, potatoes, ice creams... Yes, this is the funny part of super saturation!

Let's make a graph here to show what has happened to the level of glycogen/glucose store inside your muscles.

As you can see, on Days Six, Five, Four before the event, the level stays low, because the athlete has depleted and then, because he or she stays on a low carbohydrate diet and maintains endurance exercise, the level stays low. But, because on Days Three, Two and One before the event, huge amounts of carbohydrates are consumed and the athlete is resting, the level of glycogen/glucose stored goes quickly up to normal and then overshoots normal just before he or she participates on the day. In fact, the muscles are saturated in glycogen/glucose ready to provide the athlete with huge supplies of ATP and therefore, added energy with which to perform.

One last point. Extra glycogen stores also cause added water storage and cause muscles to gain weight. In fact, if you ever do super saturate, your muscles will feel 'heavy' or 'stiff'. I would not recommend this practice to sprinters or athletes concerned with short-term events less than 30 minutes.

The final issue in this chapter is a very important one. It is a basic concern you should know about if you are following a training programme in your gym.

How do you know exactly when you are working anaerobically or aerobically? When does the change occur? What ratios are operating during your exercise programme?

The best examples to illustrate the answer are the running events – the 100, 200 metres etc. In events up to 800 metres, which take about two and a half minutes, you can say you are working anaerobically – energy is being derived from the ATP-PC and lactic acid systems.

In events of 1000 to 4000 metres, it is true to say the energy sources are derived from all three systems, the two above and the oxygen system and that you are working anaerobically and aerobically.

In events of 4000 metres and over, 10 minutes and over (assuming you can keep going), you are working aerobically – your ATP is being produced from the oxygen system.

Now you can see why the mechanics of your aerobics class must be structured to include the 'aerobics section' (running, jumping etc.) with duration in excess of ten minutes. Otherwise, it's not aerobics, is it?

Summary

In this chapter we discussed energy, and went through the changes of energy forms, especially chemical into mechanical. Food is used to produce a high-energy chemical called ATP, which is found in muscles. When this chemical is 'broken down', energy is released which allows us to move. The energy we create inside the cells of muscles can be done via three systems. Two systems are anaerobic; they can do so without the use of oxygen, but they are inefficient.

The third system is aerobic; it requires oxygen. It is also the most efficient, but it is the slowest to 'get going'. We discussed the 'fuel (glucose) muscles' use to produce ATP and how these 'fuels' can be altered in supply (Super saturation). Activities were categorized: those of short-term high intensity were classified as 'anaerobic'; those of longer duration (longer than 10 minutes) and medium intensity were classified as 'aerobic'.

Finally, training programmes (anaerobic versus aerobic) and their ratios were broadly differentiated: that is, which systems are in use, to what extent and when.

OOO

How does Aerobic Fitness benefit your Heart and Lungs?

In the last chapter we looked at the three energy systems and their relevance to exercise. The most important system in terms of energy supply during endurance exercise is the oxygen system. The oxygen system operates only when oxygen is supplied to the cells. This chapter is about how oxygen is supplied to the cells of your body.

Before it is explained, we will have to learn a bit of anatomy (the study of the structure of the human body). The two structures connected with oxygen supply to the cells are: lungs and heart.

The Lungs

Human beings have two lungs, a right one and a left one.

As you can see from the diagram, there are many components, which together are known as the 'respiratory tract'. The upper respiratory tract consists of the nasal cavity, pharynx and larynx. (A cold is an upper respiratory infection.) The lower respiratory tract consists of trachea and bronchi (plural of bronchus) and lungs. (A common infection in this region is bronchitis). So let's find out what happens to the air once it enters your nose or mouth – actually the air primarily enters your nose, because your nose filters, heats and humidifies the air. Noses also trap bacteria and smell things! Once the air is in, it passes through the pharynx—and into the larynx. Now the larynx is really interesting because most people call this 'the voice box.'

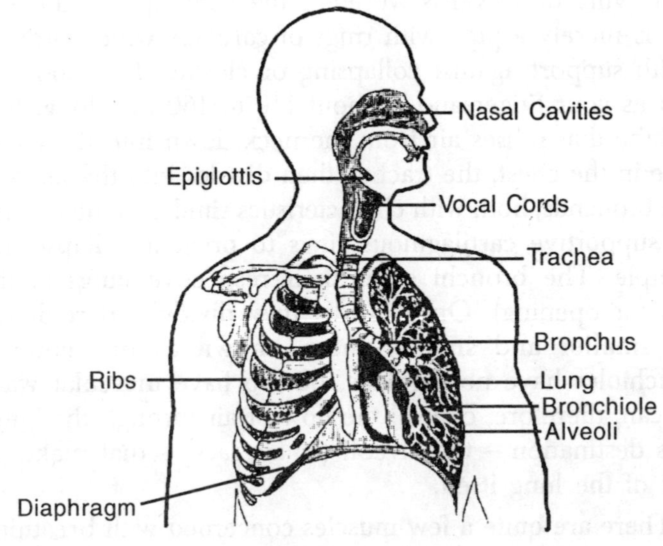

The larynx is actually a very complicated circular muscle, which surrounds the opening of the lower respiratory tract. It has quite a few cartilages (tough, white flexible tissue). One such cartilaginous structure is well known to us as the 'Adam's apple', the thyroid cartilage. When the larynx is closed, the lower respiratory tract is cut off from the system of tubes concerned with digestion (alimentary canal). This is to stop food falling down into our windpipe. Actually, this does happen sometimes, when you are talking and eating at the same time, for example, and as a consequence this food has to be removed quickly by a violent blast of air from the lungs (a cough). The cough shoots the food back into the correct channels concerned with digestion. The larynx is also concerned with speech. The air passing in and out of the lungs causes the vocal chords inside the larynx to vibrate. There are two pairs of vocal chords and the muscles of the larynx can change the tension of these chords just as a guitarist can change the tone of a guitar string by tightening or loosening the strings. By controlling the tension of the vocal chords we gain 'pitch' control over our voices.

Moving downwards we enter the windpipe or trachea. This is merely a pipe with rings of cartilage which provide it with support against collapsing or closing. It is about as thick as your finger and is about 140 to 160 mm long. It is the tube that passes air from the neck down into the chest. Once in the chest, the trachea then divides into the left and right bronchus, both with characteristics similar to the trachea and supportive cartilaginous rings to prevent collapse, for example. The bronchi enter their respective lungs at the hilus (or opening). Once inside, they divide and re-divide into smaller and smaller tubes known as bronchioles. Bronchioles have no cartilage, but do have muscular walls and can, therefore, control the flow of air through the lungs to its destination – the alveoli (or air sacs) – that make up most of the lung itself.

There are quite a few muscles concerned with breathing but it is needless to list them. It is enough to know the fact that lungs have an elastic nature and can recoil after each contraction into the relaxed position, and that the main muscle contracting under rest conditions is the diaphragm. Like a muscle sheet stretched under your ribs, the diaphragm lengthens and shortens the chest cavity, causing changes in lung volume.

Getting back to the bronchioles, while breathing in their diameter increases somewhat and allows more air to pass in. Each time one breathes out, their diameter is reduced, thereby reducing lung volume and the amount of air in them, and so you breathe out.

Normally, lungs have a pale pink colour, but if one smokes heavily they turn grey from pink. Your lungs are filled and spongy. Many people think that when they breathe in, their lungs blow up like a balloon, and when they breathe out, they collapse. What actually happens is that your lungs inflate; each breath you take makes up a portion of the total lung volume. During inhalation (breathing in) about 500 ml of air is drawn through the trachea and into the lungs. During expiration (breathing out) about 500 ml of air is expelled. This exchange of 500 ml of air in and out is known as 'tidal air'. The average person has approximately another 1 litre of residual air that is always present in the lungs, bronchi and trachea, even at rest.

The alveoli or air sacs are the really vital components of our lungs. This is where blood takes up the oxygen and carbon dioxide (waste) is given off from the blood. This whole process is known as 'gas exchange'. The lungs are divided into lobes or compartments; there are two in the left and three in the right.

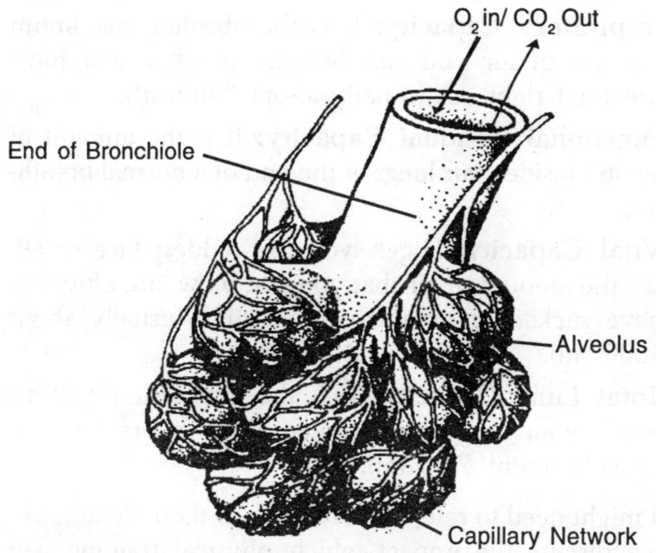

To conclude our discussion of the lungs, it is important to describe the various ways in which lung volumes can be expressed.

1. **Tidal Volume:** It is the volume of air breathed in and out with each breath (about 500 ml).
2. **Inspiratory Reserve Volume:** It is the extra amount of air you can get into your lungs (about 3000 ml)which is over and above the normal tidal air.

3. **Expiratory Reserve Volume:** It is the extra amount of air you can blow out of your lungs (usually about 1000 ml and doing which gives you a much red face) after you have expired your tidal air.
4. **Residual Volume:** It is the amount of air still left inside your lungs after the most forceful breathe-out that you can perform (usually about 1200 ml) and this gives you a very, very red face!

When we consider the effects of exercise on the lungs, we really have to consider changes in lung capacities, as well as the volumes discussed above. So let's look at lung capacities which are the norm.

1. **Inspiratory Capacity:** It is the absolute maximum amount of air you can breathe in after you have breathed right out (usually about 3500 ml).
2. **Functional Residual Capacity:** It is the amount of air still inside your lungs at the end of a normal breath-out.
3. **Vital Capacity:** It gets you the reddest face of all. It's the amount of air that you can blow out, after you have sucked in as much as possible (usually about 4600 ml).
4. **Total Lung Capacity:** It is the total amount of air inside your lungs after a huge effort of breathing in (usually about 5700 ml).

You might need to refer back later on to these definitions, when we discuss the impact which physical training will have in influencing lung capacities.

The Heart

It's a fact that the greatest cause of death in the twentieth century was heart illness. Diet, exercise, alcohol, stress, smoking, etc., all get mentioned when heart care is discussed. But again, before any sensible discussion about the heart, an understanding of its components is essential.

Your heart is about the size of your fist and is contained in an envelope called the pericardium. It can be compared to two pumps – one pump is on the left side, the other on the right. These two pumps work together, synchronized perfectly to within a split second. As you can see from the proceeding diagram, there are chambers (cavities) and valves (structures which will allow blood to flow in one direction only). The key to understanding how the heart works is to remember that blood only flows in one direction all the time. It's a one-way system and you'll have to arrive back at the start in the end, anyway.

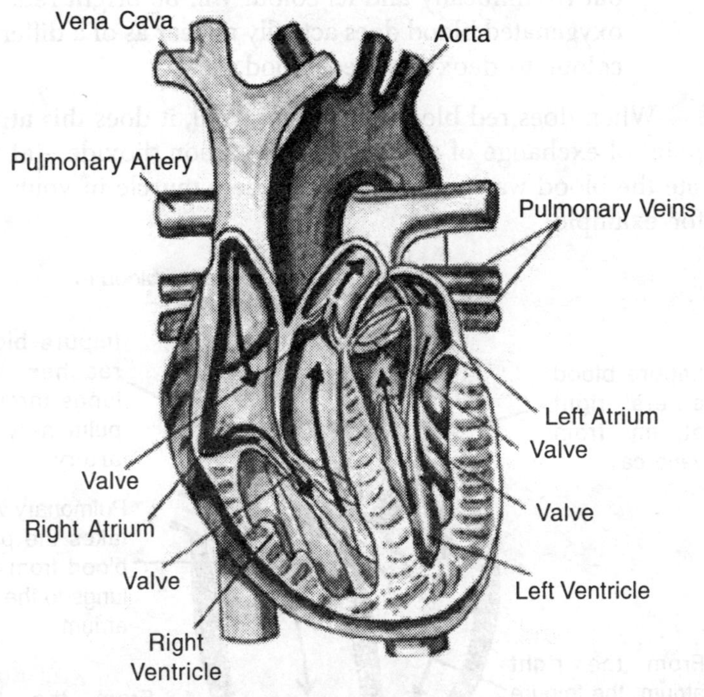

Summary

Pulmonary Circulation

Right side – de-oxygenated – blue blood

Systemic Circulation

Left side – oxygenated – red blood

Now the purpose of the heart beating is twofold:

1. Pulmonary Circulation gets blood to the lungs to pick up oxygen and get rid of carbon dioxide (waste). Blood in the right of the heart pump is known as 'blue' or deoxygenated blood. When you injure your knee or cut your finger slightly, the blue blood – actually a dull red colour – oozes out.
2. Systemic Circulation gets the blood with oxygen to all living cells in your body and collects carbon dioxide from the cells. Blood in the left heart is 'red' or oxygenated blood. If you sever an artery (because of a very deep cut to your arm, say), blood will squirt out rhythmically and its colour will be bright red. So, oxygenated blood does actually appear as of a different colour to deoxygenated blood.

When does red blood turn blue? Well, it does this at the point of exchange of oxygen for the carbon dioxide – at the site the blood was pumped to, may be a muscle in your leg, for example.

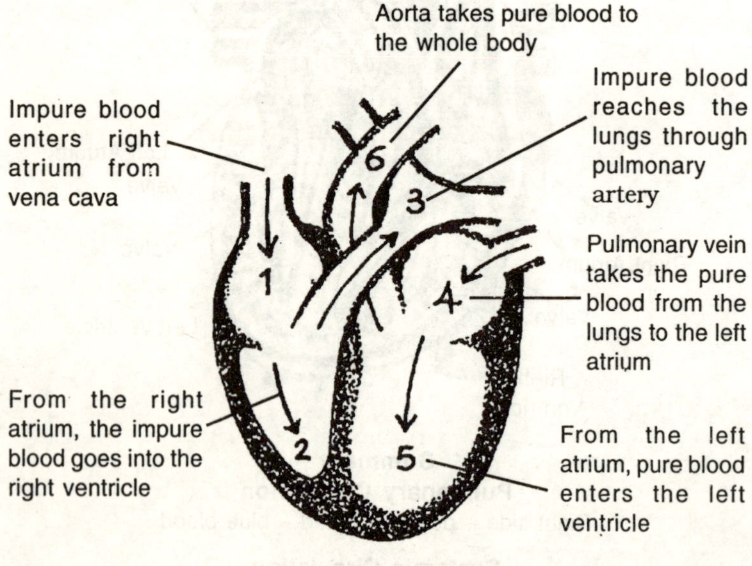

Blood Vessels

Before we discuss the pulmonary and systemic circulation pathways, let's know the following:

1. Arteries are the muscular-walled blood vessels carrying blood away from the heart.
2. Arterioles are small arteries.

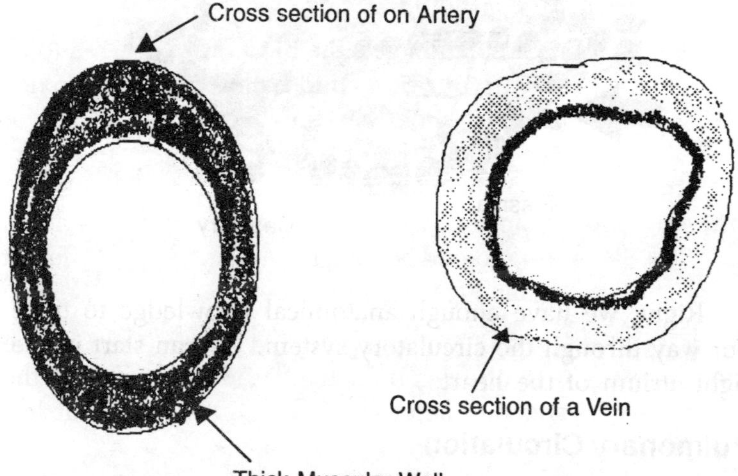

3. **Your Capillaries:** Capillaries are the smallest vessels– microscopic in size, in the circulatory system. Red blood cells actually have to travel through these vessels in a single file in many cases. This is the site where oxygen is exchanged for carbon dioxide. The substances needed by your cells pass out of your blood when it is in your capillaries. The capillary walls are only one-cell thick. Plasma and oxygen, from the red cells, are able to pass through the walls and into your tissue fluid. The tissue fluid carries the substances into the individual cells. It also carries waste products from the cells into the capillaries, or else into lymph vessels to be absorbed into the blood later via a vein.
4. Venules are small veins.
5. Veins are collapsible walls, carrying blood back to the heart.

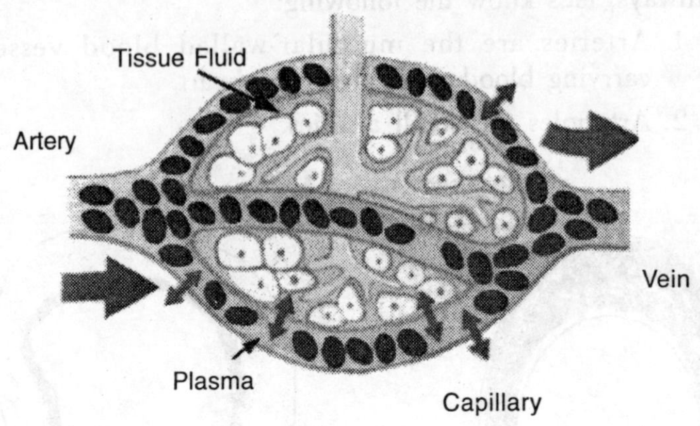

Right, we have enough anatomical knowledge to trace our way through the circulatory system. We can start in the right atrium of the heart.

Pulmonary Circulation

Blood passes in through the right atrioventricular valve (a valve made up of three flaps). Remember the heart is a muscle, and it ensures that all the blood does go into the right ventricle; to do this the atrium actually contracts thus emptying its contents into the right ventricle.

When the right ventricle is full, it too contracts and in doing so shuts the atrioventricular valve so that blood can't go back up into the right atrium. The pulmonary valve opens and the blood content of the right ventricle is squeezed into the pulmonary artery. Once the blood is in the pulmonary artery, the ventricle relaxes and the pulmonary valve shuts again, preventing blood from moving backwards. Blood is now inside the pulmonary artery and is off to the lungs, and it branches into the left and right pulmonary arteries, one to supply each lung.

Once in the lungs, the arteries divide and re-divide into a network of the tiny vessels called capillaries. These capillaries surround the alveoli (or air sacs) previously mentioned, inside the lungs. Because the alveoli are full of air, the blood is free to exchange carbon dioxide for oxygen. Having collected the vital oxygen, the blood then leaves the network of capillaries and moves on into the venules and veins to make its way from the lungs back to the heart again – freshly supplied with oxygen.

You may be asking yourself how blood 'takes up' oxygen. The way it does this is through a complex molecule found in red blood cells which contains iron (haeme) and protein (globin), called haemoglobin. This molecule is capable of combining with oxygen and when it does, it is then known as oxyhaemoglobin.

The blood heading back towards the heart with rich supplies of oxygen travels in four vessels known as the pulmonary veins: two pulmonary veins from the right lung and two from the left. All four pulmonary veins empty their contents into the left atrium.

Systemic Circulation

So the left atrium fills with oxygenated blood from the lungs. The left atrium contracts and blood passes through the left atrioventricular valve (a valve made up of two flaps) into the left ventricle.

We will go to the quadriceps muscles – the ones just above your knee – to illustrate our systemic journey further. OK, so we're inside the left ventricle. The left ventricle then contracts. Blood passes into the aorta through the aortic valve. The ventricle relaxes once all the blood has been ejected into the aorta and the aortic semilunar valve shuts to prevent backflow. As this is a huge artery, the aorta leaves the heart it arches and then travels down inside your trunk. Various branch-arteries leave the aorta (e.g. the renal artery to the kidneys etc.) until the aorta itself divides into left and right common iliac arteries. Remember, we are off to the quadriceps, so our next turn will be into the femoral artery and then finally into the network of capillaries inside the quadriceps muscles. Having exchanged the oxygen for carbon dioxide in the capillaries of the quadriceps, the blood again heads back towards the heart through the femoral vein. Then this vessel joins others to make a really large vein (corresponding in importance to the aorta) known as the inferior vena carva (the superior vena carva returns blood from the head region). The superior and inferior vena carvae finally return blood to the right atrium for another round of pulmonary and systemic circulation.

See, I told you we'd end up back at where we started!

The Cardiac Cycle

1. When the right atrium contracts, the left atrium contracts at exactly the same time.
2. When the right ventricle contracts, the left ventricle contracts at the same time.

When you visit the doctor and he listens to your heart, he hears the sounds known as 'lubb-dupp' (i.e. lubb-dupp, lubb-dupp, lubb-dupp........). The lubb sound, (loudest and first sound) is due to the slamming shut of the atrioventricular valves and the vibrations associated to this event. The dupp sound (softer and second sound) is due to the slamming shut of the aortic and pulmonary valves.

In the average person, when his heart is beating normally at rest, it beats at about 72 times per minute, just over once a second. Actually, each cycle lasts about 0.8 second. The cardiac cycle is made up of contractions called 'systole' and relaxations, 'diastole', thus:

1. **Atrial systole**: atrial contraction, 0.1 sec.
2. **Ventricular systole:** ventricular contraction, 0.3 sec.
3. **Heart diastole:** relaxation of the Atria and Ventricles, 0.4 sec.

Blood Pressure

Blood pressure is the pressure which blood applies to the walls of the blood vessels in which it is contained. Blood pressure in arteries is higher than the blood pressure in veins. Because of this the walls of arteries are always being stretched. Arterial blood pressure gets its force from the discharge of blood from the left ventricle into the aorta, which is already full of blood and which is pushed onwards. When the left ventricle contracts (ventricular systole), it pushes blood into the aorta. The event gives rise to a pressure known as systolic blood pressure. Systolic blood pressure can be measured with a **sphygmomanometer** – the thing the doctor pumps up while you wear an inflated sleeve on your arm and then lets the inflation down slowly. With the same device, you can measure diastolic blood pressure – the pressure which occurs when the heart is resting. Usually normal blood pressure (BP) in an adult is expressed like this:

$$BP = \frac{120}{80 \text{ mm Hg}}$$

120 is the systolic blood pressure; 80, the diastolic blood pressure; and pressure is measured in mm Hg, millimetres of mercury, as read off the sphygmomanometer's mercury filled tubes.

120/80 mm Hg is considered to be normal adult blood pressure, but these figures vary according to time of day, sex, age, emotional state and other factors. Blood pressure increases with age and is often higher in women than men.

Things One Should Know About Blood Pressure

There must be enough blood circulating in the vessels to maintain normal blood pressure. A good example here is when someone is seriously injured in a car accident and as a consequence, loses a lot of blood. An accompanying fall in blood pressure is the result.

Heart output is mainly measured by stroke volume. This is the amount of blood ejected each time the ventricles contract (ventricular systole). It doesn't tell the whole story. People heavily into the heart's output need to talk about force, too, but that needn't concern us here too much.

If stroke volume is increased, systolic pressure increases. The walls of arteries are elastic. Indeed, there is quite a lot of elastic material inside the artery walls, especially large arteries like the aorta. They can stand more blood being pumped–as long as they don't get hardened by lack of exercise or high fat and cholesterol diets. Increases in stroke volume cause increases in efficiency and are very good for you, as we will see later, making the circulation system work better, work more efficiently and not by working harder – quite the contrary.

How are Lungs Benefited from Aerobic Exercise?

People often ask, "What good does physical training do? As soon as you stop, you revert back to stage one, so what's the point? What do you get out of all the effort you put into physical endurance training?"

Well, let's consider changes to your breathing systems first.

An endurance fitness programme has the following effects:

1. Tidal volume is increased – more air passes in and out.
2. The whole purpose of having lungs is to allow you to consume oxygen and blow out carbon dioxide, and training causes an increase in breathing efficiency; that is, less air will be required in the lungs to obtain the same oxygen consumption that someone untrained needs – the trained individual can consume oxygen from less air than the untrained.
3. Endurance fitness training increases the various lung volumes at rest.
4. Trained people tend to have larger capacities than untrained people.
5. The larger lung volumes of trained people provide a larger surface area for the alveoli/capillary networks.

Well, there are five good reasons for sweating it out in your gym, but just wait until you see how endurance physical training affects the heart.

How is Heart Benefited from Aerobic Exercise?

We should perhaps begin with changes to the heart while resting. The very size of your heart itself changes, and the type of change varies according to the type of training programme you have followed.

From aerobic (or endurance) training you can expect the ventricular chambers of the heart to become larger, therefore, accommodating a larger volume of blood per beat of the heart. This 'volume per beat' is known as stroke volume. Also the muscular walls of your heart will become stronger and every 'beat' or 'contraction' of its muscle will increase in strength, thus pumping blood into the aorta/pulmonary arteries more efficiently every time your heart beats–over 100,000 benefits everyday.

From weight lifting (or power) training, where you are involved in maximum short-burst/heavy load types of exercise, you can expect the ventricular muscle walls of the heart to thicken. The ventricular chambers remain the same, unlike the aerobic exercisers, but the heart walls will become thicker. Each time you work at your power event the heart can beat with fast, powerful contractions and thus, provide supply to the skeletal muscles – the ones that move you around – performing the exercise. Because the ventricular chambers stay the same, stroke volume remains the same.

Enlargement of the heart is known as 'cardia hypertrophy'.

The changes above are not immediate. It may take years before the changes in heart size occur. Training, whether endurance or otherwise, must be consistent and kept at the high level. Another point: because the heart muscle has increased in size, this is accompanied by an increase in capillary density – that is to say, your heart will receive a better supply of blood, and therefore, a better supply of oxygen.

Accompanying cardia hypertrophy is a decrease in heart rate. (Remember, we are discussing the heart changes at rest.) The resting heart rate is lower in endurance-trained people than untrained people. Why? Well, the fact that stroke volume has increased and the contractile ability of the heart has also increased in trained people, is thought to be responsible for this. In endurance trained people, the heart can 'hold' more blood (ventricular chamber enlargement) during diastole, when the ventricle is relaxed. Because the heart has also generally increased in strength, it can empty the ventricles really thoroughly during ventricular systole, the ventricle contracts and therefore, more blood per stroke will be ejected into the aorta and pulmonary arteries.

So, say, your body requires about 1 litre of blood per minute to complete a specific task – to rest, for example. Say, your heart rate is 80 beats per minute. This will mean your stroke volume is 12.5 ml per beat.

$$\text{Cardiac output} = \text{Stroke volume} \times \text{heart rate/minute}$$

$$1 \text{ litre} = \text{Stroke volume} \times 80$$

$$\text{Stroke volume} = 1/80 \text{ litre} = 0.0125 \text{ litre} = 12.5 \text{ ml}$$

That example was for an untrained person. If you follow an endurance-training programme for a year or so, and do the same calculation, you can simply measure the improvement in efficiency. You will still require 1 litre of blood per minute to rest, but you take your heart rate and its lower: only 60 beats per minute!

$$\text{Cardiac output} = \text{Stroke volume} \times \text{heart rate/minute}$$

$$1 \text{ litre} = \text{Stroke volume} \times 60$$

$$\text{Stroke volume} = 1/60 \text{ litre} = 0.0166 \text{ litre} = 16.6 \text{ ml}$$

So, exercise has increased the stroke volume from 12.5 ml to 16.6 ml, and 33 per cent more blood is being pumped from your heart with every stroke. Also, your heart is now beating only 60 times per minute instead of 80 to keep you alive at rest, so it will now beat 29,000 times less often every single day than it would if you had not done the training programme.

So by following an endurance programme, you could save your heart over 10 million beats a year. For your own comparisons, the average resting heart rate in India is 72 beats per minute.

Physical training has been proven to cause increases in muscle size (muscular hypertrophy) and increases in capillary supply to muscle fibres. Each muscle fibre has a capillary supply, and this supply of capillaries can be increased by 50 per cent through physical training programmes. Consequently, oxygen and nutrient supply to the muscle are enhanced. Also, waste products from the muscle can be efficiently transported away by the bloodstream.

Both blood volume and haemoglobin levels increase with physical training programmes.

There are four more important reasons for continuing to sweat it out at your fitness centre, but just to finish on a high note, let's look at changes during maximal exercise – when you are going full bore!

Cardiac output and stroke volume are not only increased at rest. Under conditions of maximum exercise, the improvement survives. Due to the heart enlargement caused by endurance training, especially the enlargement of the ventricular chambers, the stroke volume has increased per beat, and cardiac output (= stroke volume × heart rate/m) is increased. In general, blood supply is increased.

But there is no significant change in the maximum heart rate. Most people are confused about maximum heart rates. When you exercise, as you no doubt know, your heart rate picks up almost immediately. The faster you exercise, the faster your heart goes.

How fast can it go? The range is from as little as 20 or 30 beats per minute up to as high as 250 beats per minute.

So don't be confused if endurance training doesn't increase your maximum heartbeat – you are getting the benefit in volume per stroke, not more strokes.

What causes it to beat slowly or quickly? Nerves cause it predominantly. Inside your body there are three 'separate' nervous systems. The first one you all know is voluntary *i.e.* you control it. You may decide to lift up your big left toe and your voluntary nerves will perform this task under your will. The other two systems are together known as the autonomic system. They are involuntary and there's not much you can do willingly about their behaviours! The heart is controlled by the autonomic system, which has two branches, the sympathetic and parasympathetic nervous systems. The sympathetic nervous system is sometimes called 'drive' and is responsible for increases in heart rate and heart contractile strength. The parasympathetic nervous system decreases heart rate.

Summary

So, you can now see that training in your gym or for that matter anywhere else is really worthwhile. If anyone asks you why you do it, you have a dozen really good reasons to give them. You can also see that the majority of beneficial changes to your cardio-respiratory systems are attributed to the endurance type training, aerobics. There is no easy way to achieve high levels of fitness.

By reading this and understanding the benefits of endurance exercise, I hope I have helped to convince you that exercising is a truly worthwhile pursuit.

OOO

All About Calories

So far we have discussed Aerobics (energy systems), the effects of aerobic exercise on your heart and lungs, and how to measure these effects.

So, where do calories fit in? A calorie is simply a unit of measurement; just as inches or centimetres are measurements of length, calories are simply measurement of energy.

Here's the conversion, for those studying light cans, packets of slim milk powder and breakfast foods and the like:

1 calorie = 4.2 kilojoule (kJ)
1 kilojoule = 0.24 calories

Your body creates its own energy to keep itself alive and 'moving'. To create energy in the form of human movement you have to supply your body with food and oxygen–or chemical energy. Well, the amount of chemical energy you put into your body can be measured in calories.

Well back in the 1880s, a scientist called Max Rubner invented a device called the bomb calorimeter. It consisted of a chamber (which looked a bit like a bomb) around which was circulating water. The chamber was then insulated so as to keep heat from leaving the inside. He then placed a potato in the chamber and burned it. He measured the temperature of the water and noticed that it increased. The heat energy released from the burning spud had caused the temperature of the circulating water to rise. Max decided to precisely measure the increase in water temperature for different types of food. Next he decided to burn a pizza with the entire lot the anchovies. Before 'ignition' the water temperature was 15 degree Celsius. The pizza was burned and he again measured the water temperature. It had risen to 20 degree Celsius, a rise of 5 degree Celsius. There was 100g of water circulating his Bomb Calorimeter. So, if 100g of water had received an increase of 5 degree Celsius in temperature, the temperature of 1 gram of water under the same experiment would have risen by 500 degree Celsius!

So, now you know what a calorie is. It is unit of energy which is equal to the amount of heat required to raise the temperature of one gram of water one degree Celsius. The obvious question now is how many calories do you need every day?

This is dependent upon your energy needs. When you were young, a teenager for example, you needed a lot more energy than say, after the age of 40-45. This is because teenagers and youngsters are active. They run or walk everywhere, they play sports, perform physical activities at school. But during adulthood, we slow down.

All fairly obvious, but what is it that seems to go wrong with so many people? Why do they let themselves go and get fat?

Your body is a dynamo, creating energy from food and oxygen and if too much food energy is put in, your body stores it in fat deposits on thighs, arms and bellies. Now you must remember that 'getting fat' is a slow process. You don't do it overnight. Many people get fat because of bad habits. They are used to three square meals a day, a necessity during their youth but as life goes on and life patterns change, so their food intakes should change. Eating breakfast and lunch and dinner is just too much, and they continue, regardless of bulging fat and chubby cheeks.

Another cause of 'getting fat' is an intake of too many foods which get big scores on Max's calorimeter, like greasy curries, ghee-rich food, meat – all contain hundreds of calories and if you eat them regularly, you will notice gains in weight and fat.

Excess of fat is related to a number of diseases, including diabetes, coronary heart disease, kidney disease, hypertension and several more.

We all know that being really fat isn't the best, but what can we do about it? There are many commercial facilities and fads relating to weight loss but the way to maintain a sensible approach towards weight control is through an understanding of the mechanics of calorie expenditure versus calorie intake.

Calorie Expenditure

We know what calories are and how they are determined. So first let's look at calorie expenditure. This is the number of calories you use or burn up. How many calories you use per day is going to depend upon the amount of physical activity you complete each day.

There are averages of course, depending on age: approximately 2500 to 2800 calories per day for men under 40, and 2200 to 2500 for women; and 2000 to 2300 for men aged 40 plus, and 1800 to 2000 for women.

I did say 'Averages'. There are activities you can participate in to make radical changes to those figures. Here are few examples of calorie burning (values approximate):

One hour of:	
Dancing	320 calories
Football	500
Running	700
Tennis	400
Skiing	750
Swimming	700-800
Squash	600
Golf	350
Aerobics	
Beginners	320
Intermediate	450
Advanced	600-700

So, participation in the above activities can influence daily average calorie expenditure significantly.

Calorie expenditure is somewhat more difficult to calculate daily as you are involved in such different movements/activities from hour to hour, so here is a guide to calorie expenditure for various everyday activities that most people might complete in an average day:

Sleep–About 6 calories per hour

Sitting–About 100 calories per hour

Eating, watching TV, sewing, passive sitting–About 120 calories per hour

Driving–About 150 calories per hour

Standing–About 150 calories per hour

Performing light activities (dusting, dish-washing etc.) – About 150 calories per hour

Walking fast–About 300 calories per hour

Walking upstairs–About 1000 calories per hour

Running–About 700 calories per hour

So you can use the list above and get a fairly accurate idea of how many calories you are burning in a day.

Getting fat is a gradual process; it takes place over a period of years. Weight loss is also gradual, not years, but it may take some months before your target weight is reached.

Calorie Intake

Calorie intake is the amount of energy you receive each day from foods. Now I could prepare a huge list of all the various food types and the calories contained therein, but I won't. There are heaps of well-prepared books with calorie intake values everywhere. The purpose of this chapter is to provide you with an understanding of how to manipulate these two components of weight control (calorie expenditure versus calorie intake) to achieve your correct weight.

What exactly is your correct weight? Here is a rough guide. There will obviously be some inaccuracy, but let's say an allowance of plus or minus 1.5 kg per category will be wise.

Height	Men	Women
150cms (5')	52kg	48kg
157cms (5'-2")	56kg	52kg
162cms (5'-4")	60kg	55kg
167cms (5'-6")	64kg	59kg
172cms (5'-8")	68kg	61.5kg
177cms (5'-9")	71kg	64.8kg
182cms (6')	76kg	68.5kg
188cms (6'-2")	79kg	72.0kg
193cms (6'-4")	83kg	72.5kg

If you want to lose weight, you have to decrease your intake of calories and increase your physical activity or calorie expenditure.

Here's how we do it. Get two sheets of paper, one entitled **'Calorie Intake'** (Food energy) and the other sheet entitled **'Calorie Expenditure'**.

Week 1: You just follow a normal average week. Do not alter your physical activity pattern. Write down under Monday, Tuesday etc. your details on each sheet every night. Be as accurate as possible. Calorie values are available from any calorie guide or weight-watching manual. Add them up for each day.

Week 2: You prepare two fresh sheets, one for calorie intake, the other for calorie expenditure. Look at your sheets from Week 1. You should be able to make out what is wrong with your control over your weight. Compare each day, having totaled the calorie expenditure and calorie intakes for each day. Let's take Monday as an example: remember readings are approximate.

Calorie Expenditure Sheet – Monday Week 1

Work out calorie expenditure per hour, thus:

8 AM	Drove to work	150 Calorie
9 AM	Sat in office	100 Calorie
10 AM	Ditto	100 Calorie
11 AM	Ditto	100 Calorie
12 noon	Ditto	100 Calorie
1 PM	Sat eating lunch	100 Calorie
2 PM	Sat in office	100 Calorie
3 PM	Ditto	100 Calorie
4 PM	Ditto	100 Calorie
5 PM	Ditto	100 Calorie
6 PM	Ditto	100 Calorie
7 PM	Drove Home	150 Calorie
8 PM	Dinner	100 Calorie
9 PM	TV	100 Calorie
10 PM	Ditto	100 Calorie
11 PM	Bed	100 Calorie
		1700 Calorie
Sleep	60 calories × 8 hrs =	480 Calorie
Calories expended		2180 Calorie

Calorie Intake Sheet – Monday Week 1

Breakfast	1 cup coffee and butter toast and egg	380 Calorie
Morning break	1 cup tea and biscuits	250 Calorie
Lunch	Rice, vegetables, dal	1600 Calorie
Afternoon break	2 biscuits and 1 cup tea	200 Calorie
Dinner	3 chapattis, dal, vegetables, (or meat/fish)	1800 Calorie

(We Indians have the habit of having heavy dinner)

Snacks while watching TV	1 cup tea and chips, pop corn, etc.	450 Calorie

So for Monday

Total Intake	=	4680 Calorie
Less Calorie Expenditure	=	2180 Calorie
Net gain	=	2500 Calorie

The result is bad news. You will have gained weight from this imbalance of calorie expenditure vs. calorie intake.

1.

energy (calorie intake) (calorie expenditure)

food ———————————— physical activity

The Scale is balanced, so you won't get fatter, you won't get thinner!

2.

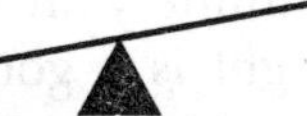

The Scale is unbalanced–calorie intake exceeds calorie expenditure, so you will get fatter.

3.

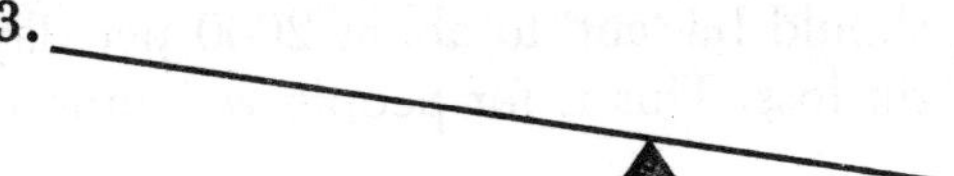

The Scale is unbalanced again–calorie expenditure exceeds calorie intake, so this time you'll get thinner!

So, back to your fresh sheets neatly headed 'Week 2' and we'll make the necessary adjustments. Let's say there's not too much you can do about the calorie expenditure for Monday, you have no time to increase physical activity: sitting and working on the computer is how you earn your money in this example. So leave calorie expenditure at 2180 calories.

Calorie intake (food energy) is where our adjustment will be made. The beauty of a self-engineered diet is that you will be able to eat the foods you enjoy eating. You don't have to live like a rabbit either. There are many foods available to you other than just lettuce. Often these foods are better for you as well, because many low calorie foods contain less cholesterol, less fat and more fibre. You won't be hungry because you can eat lower calorie foods.

Right, go through your sheets day by day and design meals for breakfast, lunch and dinner which, when their calories are added together, will be lower than your daily calorie expenditure totals, i.e. less than 2180 calories on Monday. **(I have enclosed two such sheets at the end of this chapter.)**

Make sure that when you do design your diet, you include plenty of green vegetables (fibre), grain breads or chapattis, fruits, fish, liver and high protein milk. Remove alcohol (it's fattening anyway) and try to leave sugar out of coffee and tea. Be organized. Programme your two sheets once a week for 12 weeks. Sunday night is a good time to do it.

How many calories should you take in?

1. If your Calorie Expenditure sheet from Week 1 reads around the 4000 calories a day mark, your calorie intake plan should be 'cut' to about 2000 per day to achieve weight loss. This is for people weighing over 85 kg.
2. If your Calorie Expenditure sheet from Week 1 reads around 2000-3000 calories a day mark, your calorie intake plan should be 'cut' to about 1200 calories per day for people weighing about 62 to 76 kg to achieve weight loss.
3. If your Calorie Expenditure sheet from Week 1 reads around 1500-1800 calories a day mark, your calorie intake plan should be 'cut' to about 900 calories per day for people weighing approximately 55 to 60 kg.

(Remember we are discussing weight loss here. If you need to gain weight, just do the opposite, increase the calorie intake.)

'Time' is always the problem when people try to raise their calorie expenditure, because they often are just too busy to find time to exercise. I always find this somewhat difficult to understand because I consider my life in terms of priorities, and there are only really two important things in my life: my family and health.

And if you are fortunate enough to have both, you should surely spend the time needed to look after them.

OOO

Initial Calorie Intake Chart
Duration: 7 days
(SAMPLE)
(First day has been filled as an example)

Name: Mr. Y

Sex: Male Age: 24

Introductory body weight: 72 Kg

	Mon	Tues	Wed	Thu	Fri	Sat	Sun
Breakfast	380						
Morning Tea	250						
Lunch	1600						
Afternoon	100						
Dinner	1800						
Snacks while watching TV	150						
Total	4280						

Initial Calorie Expenditure Chart

Duration: 7 days

(SAMPLE)

(First day has been filled as an example)

Name: Mr. Y

Sex: Male Age: 24

Introductory body weight: 72 Kg

	Mon	Tues	Wed	Thu	Fri	Sat	Sun
8.00 AM	250						
9.00 AM	200						
10.00 AM	200						
11.00 AM	200						
12.00 NOON	200						
1.00 PM	200						
2.00 PM	200						
3.00 PM	200						
4.00 PM	200						
5.00 PM	200						
6.00 PM	200						
7.00 PM	250						
8.00 PM	300						
9.00 PM	250						
10.00 PM	400						
11.00 PM	400						
12.00 MIDNT	480						
Total (around)	4500						

Calories Expended During Exercise

The number of calories you burn depends upon your weight, the activity you are doing and the intensity level you are exercising at. Any activity that you perform can be done at a variety of intensity levels. If you exercise at a higher intensity level, you will be working harder, expending more energy and burning more calories than someone who is not working quite so hard.

I've included four separate Activity/Calorie tables. The tables should be used as a general guideline (the numbers are approximations). The number of calories you actually burn could be slightly higher or lower, depending upon your intensity level and your weight.

The first table deals with step aerobics only. Calories are calculated for different step heights based upon a stepping rate of 120 beats per minute for a 120-pound person. If you weigh more than 120 or you are in a faster paced step class, the number of calories you'll burn will be higher than those displayed in the table. If you weigh less than 120 or you are in a slower paced step class, you'll burn fewer calories than indicated in the table. The table is just an approximation of the number of calories you expend. If you work at a more intense level (raise your arms above your shoulders, lift your knees all the way to your chest etc...) you will burn more calories than displayed. (Data for this table was taken from Reebok Instructor News, Volume 4, Number 3.)

Step Height	Calories/ min.	Calories/ 10 min.	Calories/ 30 min.
4 inches	4.5	45	135
6 inches	5.5	55	165
8 inches	6.4	64	192
10 inches	7.2	72	216

The second table gives the caloric expenditure after 10 minutes of activity for various body weights. This data was obtained from Reebok Instructor News, Volume 4, Number 2. **(2.2 pounds (lbs) = 1 kg)**

Activity & Calories /10 min.	125 lbs	150 lbs	175 lbs	200 lbs
Aerobics (traditional at high intensity)	95	115	134	153
Gardening	41	49	57	65
Racquetball	75	90	105	120
Running (9 min/mile)	109	131	153	174
Shopping	35	42	49	56
Sitting (reading or watching TV)	10	12	14	16
Sleeping	10	12	14	16
Standing (light activity)	20	24	28	32
Volleyball	28	34	40	45
Walking (15 min/mile)	44	52	61	70
Walking upstairs	150	175	202	229

The third table lists a wide variety of exercises and the caloric expenditures for a 123-lb woman and a 170-lb man.

Data for this table was taken from Reebok Instructor News, Volume 5, Number 2.

Activity & Calories /10 min.	123-lb woman	170-lb man
Basketball	77	106
Cycling (5.5 mph)	36	49
Cycling (9.4 mph)	56	74
Cycling (racing)	95	130
Dance Exercise (High Impact Aerobics)	94	124
Dance Exercise (Low Impact Aerobics)	80	105
Football	74	102
Racquetball	76	107
Rope Skipping (slow)	82	116
Rope Skipping (fast)	100	142
Running (8 min/mile)	113	150
Running (11 1/2 min/mile)	76	100
Skiing (Cross country)	80	106
Stairmaster	88	122
Step Aerobics (4 inch bench)	48	66
Step Aerobics (6 inch bench)	58	80
Step Aerobics (8 inch bench)	67	92
Step Aerobics (10 inch bench)	75	104
Soccer	78	107
Swimming (back stroke)	95	130
Swimming (breast stroke)	91	125
Swimming (fast crawl)	87	120
Swimming (slow crawl)	95	130
Swimming (side stroke)	68	90
Swimming (treading water)	35	48
Tennis (singles)	61	81
Volleyball	28	39
Weight training (super circuit)	104	137
Weight training (muscular strength)	44	60
Weight training (muscular endurance)	58	80
Walking (3.5 mph)	45	59

The last table displayed below is taken from ACE Fitness Matters, Volume 1, Number 4. Calories are given for 1 minute of activity. To determine approximately how many calories you burn in 1/2 hour. Find the activity and your weight, then multiply the number displayed by 30. If you want to lose weight, try to burn 300 calories per exercise session.

Activity & Calories/Min.	**120 lbs**	**140 lbs**	**160 lbs**	**180 lbs**
Aerobics (Traditional)	7.4	8.6	9.8	11.1
Basketball	7.5	8.8	10.0	11.3
Bowling	1.2	1.4	1.6	1.9
Cycling (10 mph)	5.5	6.4	7.3	8.2
Golf (pull/carry clubs)	4.6	5.4	6.2	7.0
Golf (power cart)	2.1	2.5	2.8	3.2
Hiking	4.5	5.2	6.0	6.7
Jogging	9.3	10.8	12.4	13.9
Running	11.4	13.2	15.1	17.0
Sitting Quietly	1.2	1.3	1.5	1.7
Skating (ice and roller)	5.9	6.9	7.9	8.8
Skiing (cross country)	7.5	8.8	10.0	11.3
Skiing (downhill and water)	5.7	6.6	7.6	8.5
Swimming (crawl and moderate pace)	7.8	9.0	10.3	11.6
Tennis	6.0	6.9	7.9	8.9
Walking	6.5	7.6	8.7	9.7
Weight Training	6.6	7.6	8.7	9.8

Cardio Equipment and Calories Burned

Just a word of warning regarding cardio equipment and calories burned. Many cardio machines don't ask for your weight and tell you that you're burning X number of calories.

The number displayed is for a person of average weight (usual average is 150 pounds). For many people, the number of calories is overstated. So, if the machine doesn't have you input your weight, don't believe the number of calories displayed.

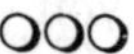

The Gymnasium Trimmings

This chapter is about 'trimmings' offered by gyms, things like spas, saunas, solariums and the like. We'll look at each one in turn.

SPAs

The main purpose of having a spa bath is to relax. The feeling of bubbling warm water against your skin is very pleasant. Some people love it. Good. But spas do nothing to increase fitness levels.

Many people are a bit skeptical about spas. They feel at risk, that they may become victims of the bacteria and germs that spas may harbour.

The truth is that if a spa is correctly maintained, the water in the spa cannot support bacterial life. In fact, the chemicals in the water of a public spa are quite strong. The chemicals used are chlorine, bromine (only recently put into spas) and hydrochloric acid. The chlorine kills bacteria, bromine also kills bacteria, and to some extent, reduces the globules of body fat which accumulate and float on the water surface, but even when bromine is placed in the spa, the rings of body fat, which still persist, should be scrubbed off the walls of the spa every two or three days. The hydrochloric acid is added to control the acidity or alkalinity of the water.

The spa should be backwashed and filtered daily.

Most commercial gyms will advise against eating or drinking in the spas for obvious reasons. The water temperature should be carefully monitored and if it is quite high, it is inadvisable to stay in it for too long. People with sensitive skin, skin irritations or open cuts or abrasions are also advised to avoid public spas.

Saunas

I have visited a lot of gyms in our country and checked out their temperatures in the saunas, those wood-lined hot rooms where people sit and sweat. In most cases the temperature gauges were broken, but the control knobs on the outside wall were always twisted to 'Max'. The temperature when at maximum in a sauna (and the door is kept closed) ranges from 100°C to 110°C (212°F and 220°F). This is positively dangerous. They have no fitness benefits at all; skin improvements claimed are, at best, dubious.

Your body temperature is 37°C (98.6°F) and the body goes to great effort to maintain that exact temperature all the time. Body temperature is important. If it drops, say to 36°C, you will immediately feel ill–very ill. If, on the other hand, it rises, say to 38°C, you will also feel rather ill.

If you place a human machine which maintains an accurate operating temperature into an environment three times normal environmental temperature, you are quite simply causing the 'machine' to overheat.

Your body is continuously producing heat as a by-product of metabolism, the chemical reactions occurring within your body. There are four methods by which heat is lost from your body. All four methods become less effective from about 54°C (130°F) and above. At about 71°C (160°F) all four mechanisms are almost completely inoperative. The four mechanisms of body heat loss are:

1. **Evaporation:** This mechanism–sweating–is the main way the heat is lost during exercise. When you work or exercise at high levels of intensity, your body will be cooled only if the sweat on your skin can evaporate. In a sauna sweat does not evaporate–it just drips down onto the floor–and so no cooling of your body takes place.

2. **Radiation:** The molecules within your body are always vibrating and because of this, heat (in the form of infra-red heat rays) is continuously given off. When you are seated in a room you radiate heat away from your body to the walls of the room. At the same time, the walls of the room radiate heat towards you. If the walls of a room around you are warm (like in a sauna) they will radiate heat at you at a greater rate than you radiate heat away. So, in a sauna, radiation becomes inoperative.
3. **Conduction:** This is the transfer of heat between two objects of different temperatures, which are in contact with one another. Heat flows from warm to cool bodies. Once the temperature of the air next to your skin equals the temperature of your skin, no further body heat can be lost in this way.
4. **Convection:** The movement of air (like that given off from a fan) is known as convection. As body heat must first be conducted to the air, before the heat can be carried away in air currents, this mechanism doesn't work in a sauna.

There is one other way your body can attempt to rid itself of excessive heat: heat transfer from the inner parts of your body.

In extremely high temperatures blood flow is increased, and as a consequence, blood can be directed towards the skin (near body surface) away from the internal organs. This change in blood flow carries heat away from the body 'core' to the skin. The skin then acts as a kind of radiator to eliminate heat through conduction and convection. Unfortunately, this last part of the system simply cannot happen when you sit in a sauna.

Heat conduction away from your body can only occur when the surrounding environment is cooler than body temperature.

Things are beginning to look sad, aren't they? There you are sitting in temperatures around boiling point–there is no way for your body to keep itself cool. So what happens next?

Well, profuse sweating occurs. Your body doesn't give up easily, it just keeps applying the only mechanisms it has against this heat attack, and so you sweat merrily away! Drip, drip. Eventually, you lose quite a bit of body water.

A lot of people think sweating like this is great because they will lose weight. Wrong! Loss of body water leads to a decrease in blood volume. You actually end up having less blood in your circulatory system. After a while, your sweating rate will decrease–your body will only allow blood volume to fall to a certain level. This leads to added circulatory strain and if you don't get out of the sauna, circulatory collapse would eventually follow. You don't lose weight from this assault, because, as soon as you drink fluid, blood volume is restored to normal and the fluid you lost is immediately replaced. The salts you lost are also replaced from your diet or drinks prepared specifically to replace lost salts.

I have actually seen people performing push-ups, squats and sit-ups in saunas because they think they'll lose more weight by doing exercises in excessive heat. Facts are facts, and if you are frequently using the sauna technique to lose weight, you are wasting your time. If you really want to lose weight, only diet and exercise will do it for you. (Sorry, I don't like to mince my words).

Sitting around in saunas is not recommended for people with heart illness or associated disorders, and little wonder when you consider the huge strain placed upon the cardiovascular system in environments with temperature exceeding 70°C.

My conclusion on saunas–and steam-bath houses, too–is this: if you want to subject your body to heat stress with the risk of heart attack, and lose vital fluids from your body under the false impression of weight loss–go ahead.

As you have no doubt gathered, I'm not enthusiastic about gymnasium trimmings. When you spend your money in a gymnasium, you are making an investment in your fitness and surely you want to witness an improvement.

OOO

Warming Up and Cooling Down

Why is Warming Up Important?

To be safe, an aerobic programme should begin with a warm up period. The main purpose of warming up is to increase your heart rate slightly. This has two benefits: 1) it raises your core body temperature; and 2) it increases the blood (oxygen) flow to your muscles to prepare your body for more vigorous physical activity. Your muscles and tendons (which attach your muscles to your bones) will be more flexible for stretching after mild movement has raised your internal body temperature. This flexibility helps you increase the range of motion of your joints and may help you avoid injuries such as muscle tears and pulls.

What Muscles should I warm up?

Focus on warming up large muscle groups (i.e. quadriceps, calves, chest, etc...). In an aerobic class, participants march in place, parks, do knee lifts etc... for the legs. To warm up the chest and shoulder area, participants do shoulder rolls, arm circles etc... Runners/joggers could begin their run with a fast walk for 3 to 5 minutes followed by a stretch prior to the actual run itself.

How Long should I Warm Up?

It takes your body approximately 3 minutes to realize it needs to pump more blood to your muscles. Warm-ups should last approximately 5-10 minutes and they should incorporate stretching of large muscle groups (such as the quadriceps, calves, hamstrings, hip flexors, shoulders etc...)

Why Cool Down?

After you've reached and maintained your training heart rate level in the aerobic portion of your class, it is important to recover gently. The cool down serves two purposes: 1) it reduces your pulse; and 2) it returns the blood to your heart in sufficient quantities to rid the muscles of lactic acid (a chemical result of muscular fatigue). If you stop suddenly, the blood will pool in your legs instead of returning to your heart. Dizziness, nausea and a "worn-out" feeling are common symptoms of an improper cool down.

Duration of Cool Downs

It takes your body approximately 3 minutes to realize it does not need to pump all the additional blood to your muscles. A safe cool down period is at least 3 minutes, preferably 4-5 minutes. All cool downs should be followed by stretching of the muscles to avoid soreness and tightness.

OOO

Roy's Basic Fitness Programme

Basic fitness programme for both reducing weight and gaining weight (lean muscle weight) is based on simple exercises and training schedules. Both the schedules are for six months and are to be followed continuously without any break except for sickness and other unavoidable circumstances.

Charts have been given along with the training schedules which will help the reader chart his or her progress. The training schedules have been divided into three sections: Warm-up, Training programme and cool down.

Note: *These training programmes cannot alone produce the desired effect unless the diet programme is also strictly followed. So let's begin!*

Programme for Reducing Weight

For knowing the height-weight ratio you can look back to the previous chapters. But remember, the weights I have given are not a law that you have to follow like the Ten Commandments. Weight basically depends on your body frame or structure, so you can take it as +1 to 2 kg to the weights specified by me. And remember, a lean man can weigh as much as a fat-looking man. The lean man's weight will consist of lean muscle with very less percentage of fat. And the fat man's weight will be due to fat tissues and not lean muscles.

Training Schedules and Charts

The training schedules consist of charts and diagrams which will help you in achieving your objective, but this is only possible with determination, hard work and discipline. You can photocopy the chart given here and use it continuously for six months to be followed by more serious training schedules.

Warm Up

Warm-up is a serious matter. If you skip a warm-up and straightaway jump into the main training schedule, there are possibilities that you will incur injuries. A warm-up increases the blood flow and should be done every time before any exercise schedule. And for obese and inactive people it is even more important.

Warm Up Exercises

1. Spot Jogging (10 minutes): Stand upright and start to jog on the same spot while maintaining the same speed. Do not overdo it. Be comfortable and breathe normally.

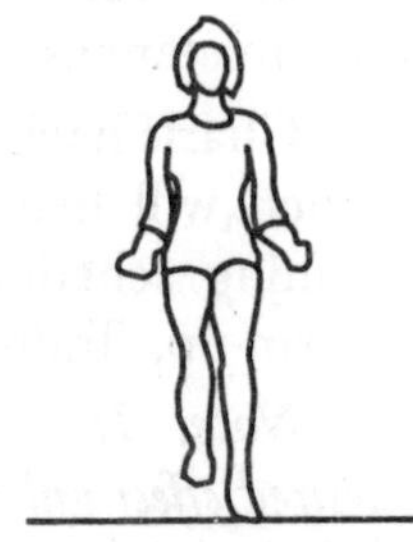

2. Jumping Jack (20 times) : Stand upright and then spread both your arms and feet at the same time. Go back to the previous posture. Breathe normally.

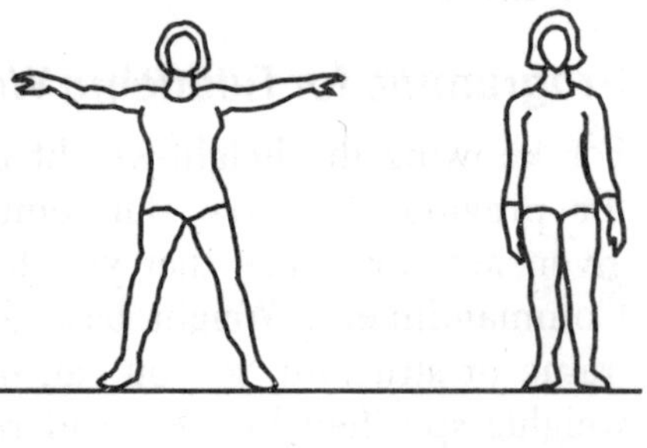

Note: *If your physical condition is such that 10 minutes of spot jogging and 20 times Jumping Jack renders you breathless, then you can decrease them to 5 minutes and 10 times respectively. The idea here is to warm up your body and increase the blood circulation, not to be out of breath and energy.*

Training Programme

Joint Movements

Head Rotation (5 Times on Each Direction)

Stand upright with your hands on your hip and rotate your head (make circles with your head) clockwise and anticlockwise. Maintain normal breathing. Never hold your breath.

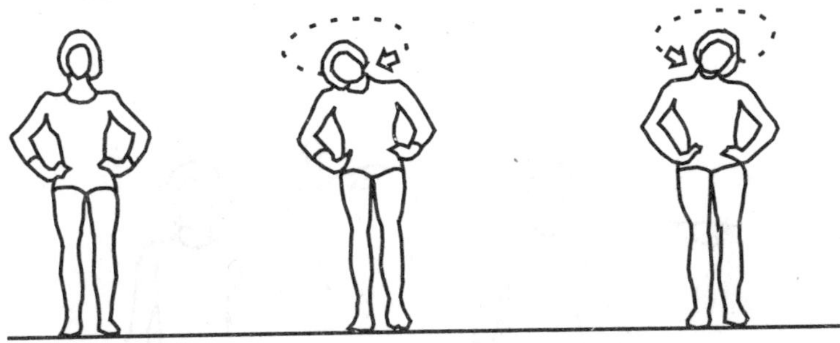

Shoulder Rotation (30 Times)

Stand upright and stretch out your right arm and make circles with it. Repeat the same with your left arm. Now stretch out both your arms and make circles with them clockwise and anticlockwise. Maintain normal breathing.

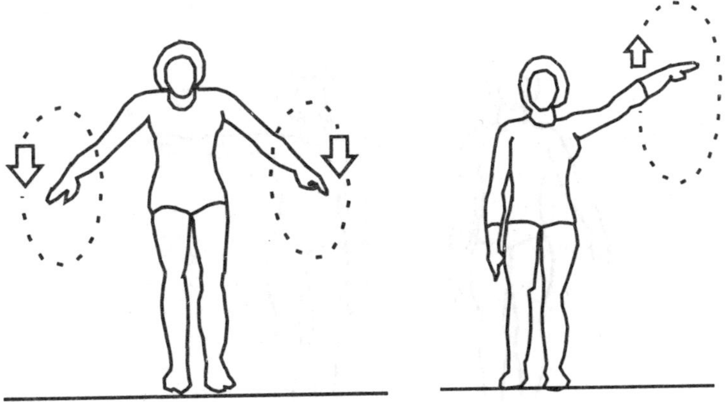

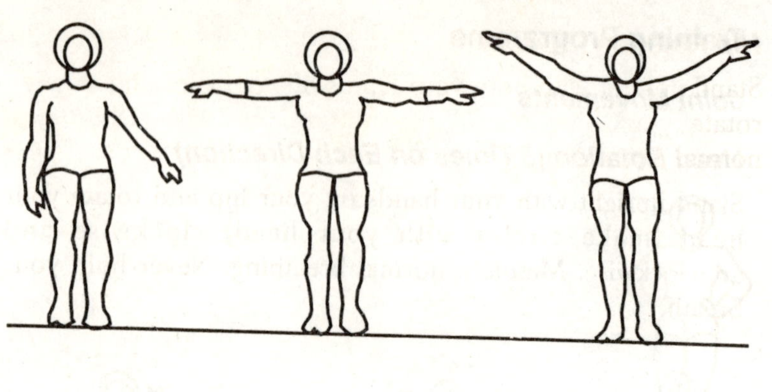

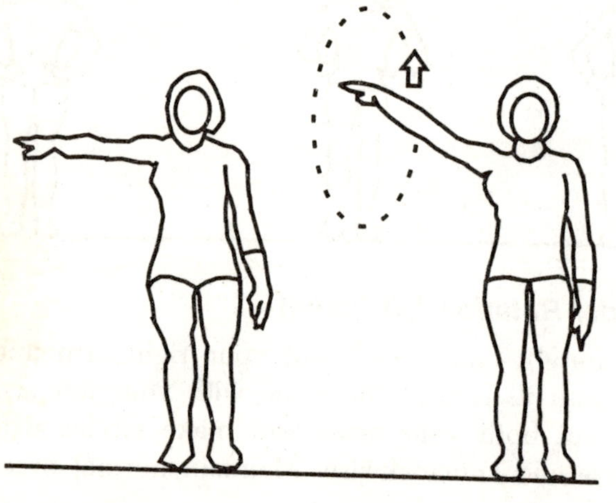

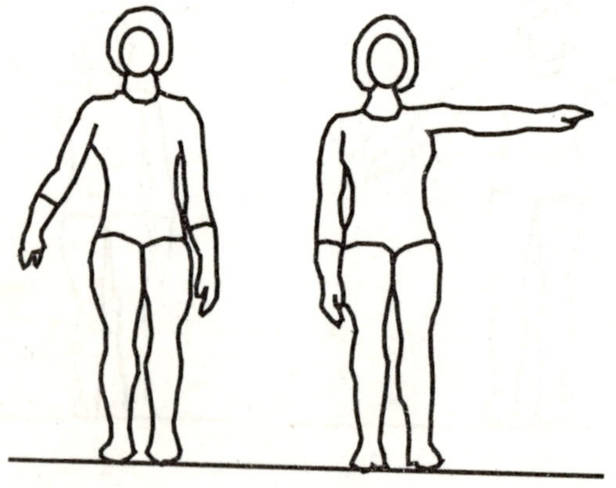

Hip Rotation (30 Times)

Stand upright with both your hands on your hips and slowly rotate your hips clockwise and anticlockwise. Maintain normal breathing.

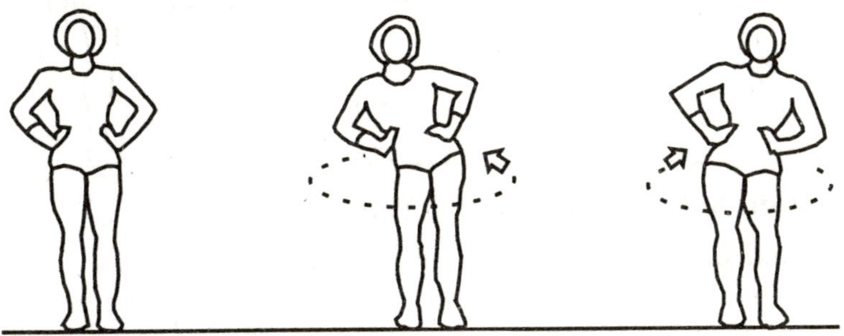

Knee Rotation (30 Times)

Bend on your knees and put both your hands on your knees. Slowly rotate your knee clockwise and anticlockwise. This at first might be a bit awkward movement for you but regular practice will remove that feeling of awkwardness.

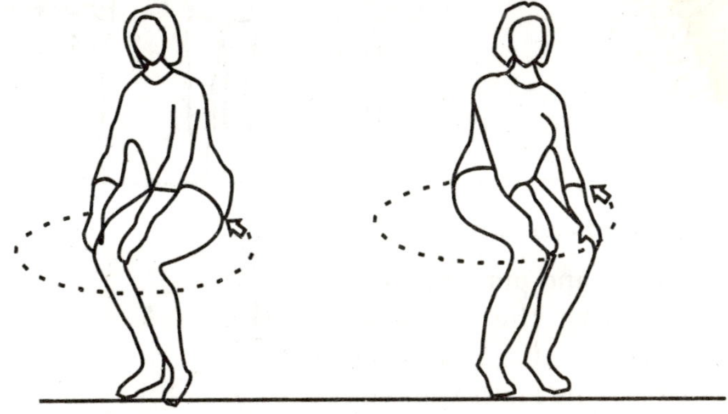

Ankle Rotation (30 Times)

Raise your right foot above the ground and rotate the ankle in the clockwise and anticlockwise directions. And then repeat it with your left leg. You may find it difficult to maintain posture but continuous practice will later make it easy.

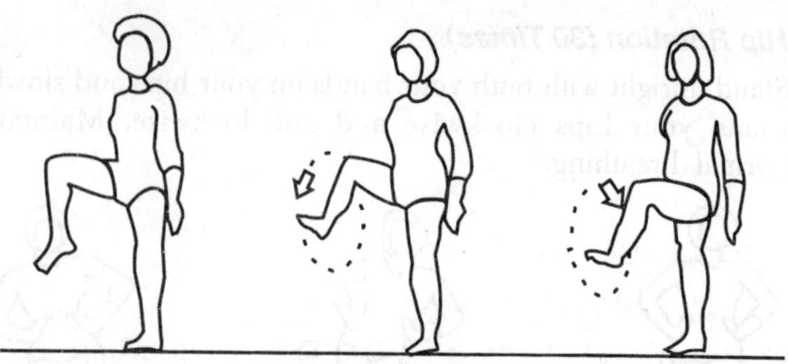

Stretching-Side Bends (20 Times)

Stand upright; put your right hand on your hip. Take your left hand on top of your head and bend towards your right. Stretch as far as you can. Repeat in the same manner on the other side.

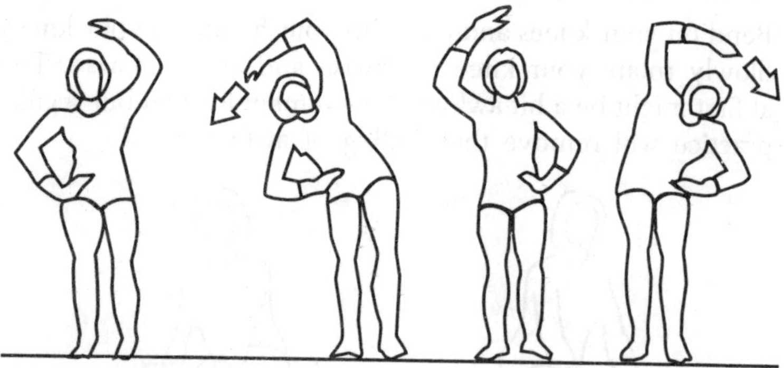

Front Bends (5 Times)

Bend down and put both your hands above the ankle as shown in the diagram. Then try to touch the knees with you head. This is a bit difficult for a novice but practice makes a man perfect!

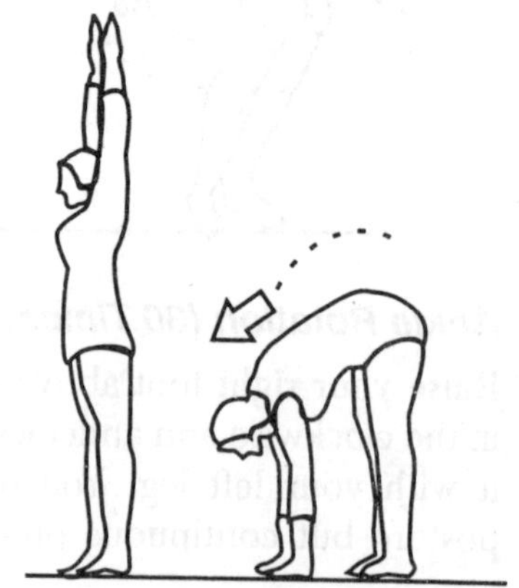

Lunges (5 Times)

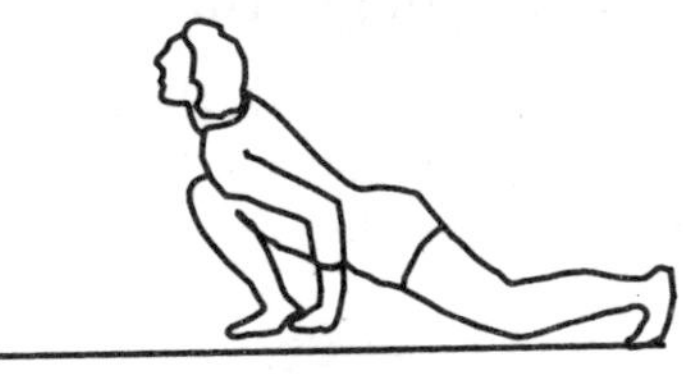

Take your right leg back so that the knee touches the floor while the left leg is bent as shown in the diagram. Repeat the exercise with the other foot.

Back Bends (3 Times)

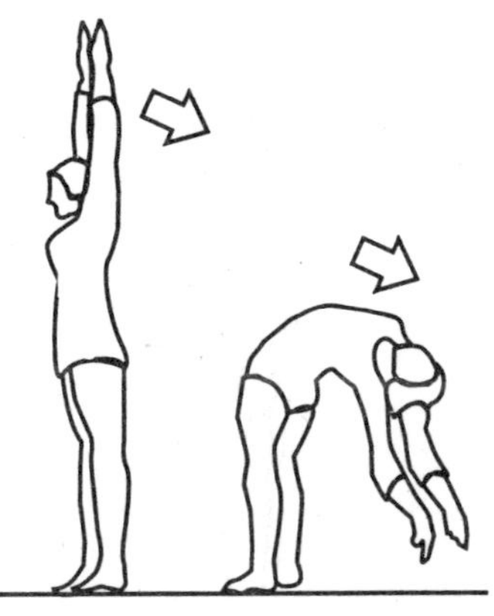

Stand upright with your hands on your hips or stretched up. Bend towards your back as if trying to touch the ground with your head. Repeat the movement three times.

Squats (20 Times)

Sit down bending your knees but remember your hips should not touch your hamstring muscles (back portion of your thighs). Do this in a rhythmic and continuous motion.

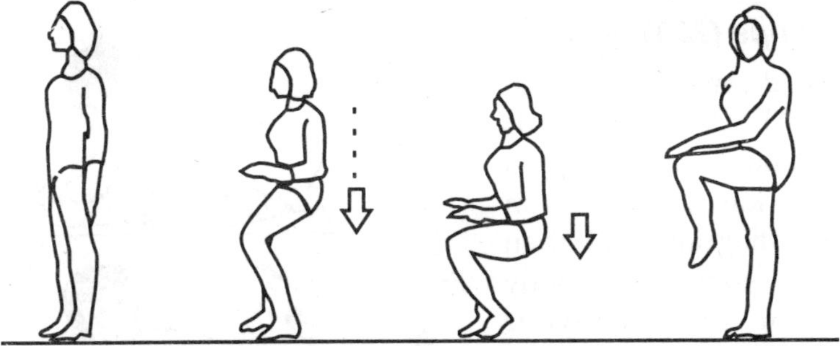

Dips (20 Times)

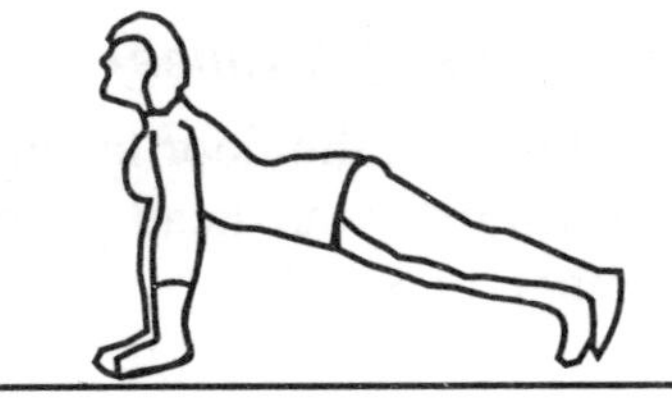

Lie down facing the floor with your palms and the toe touching the floor. Raise your chest and upper body by straightening up your arms. Repeat this twenty times.

Spot Jogging (with Hand Touching the Knees)

Stand upright and start to jog. Bring out your palms before your knees and try to touch them with your palms. Do this for 20 minutes.

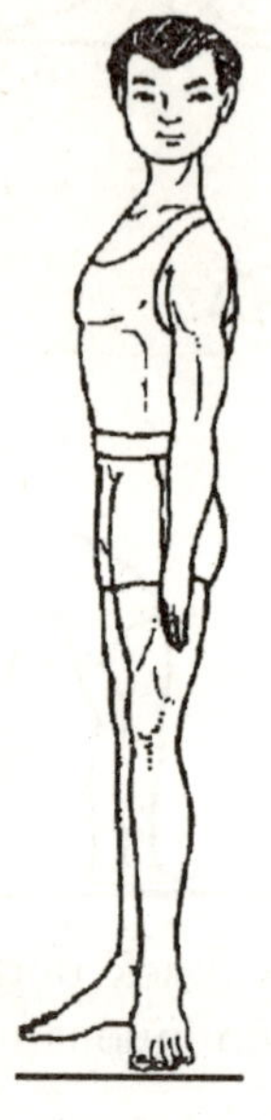

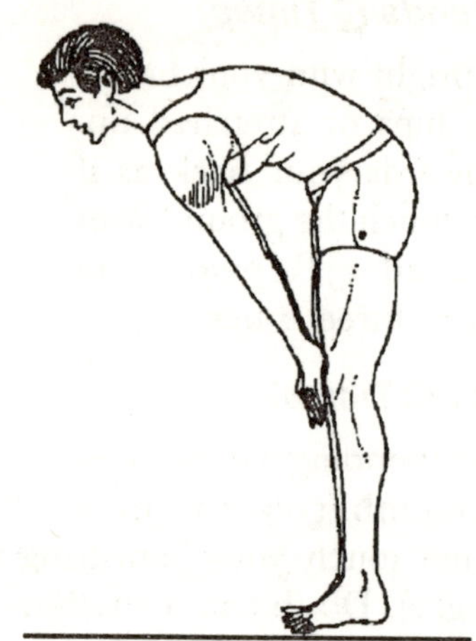

Sit-ups (20 Times)

Lie down on the floor. Put both your hands behind your neck. Bend your knees as shown in the diagram and then raise your upper body trying to touch your knees with your head. Repeat it 20 times.

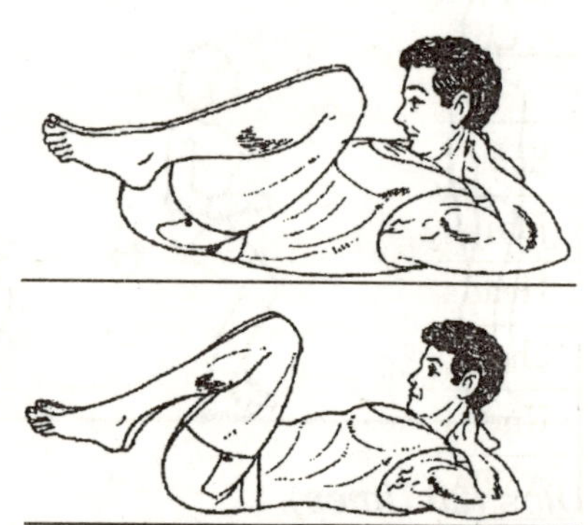

Leg Raises (20 Times)

Lie down on the floor facing the sky. Slowly raise both your feet towards your head. Repeat the movement for specified number of times.

Cool Down

As warm up is important, cool down is also important. It brings back the body temperature and circulation back to normal.

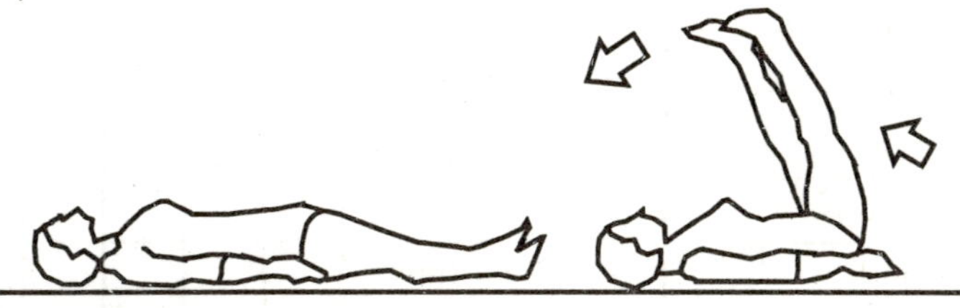

Vacuum (15 Times)

Stand upright. Take a deep breath and blow out your stomach as if it becomes a pumped balloon. Then breathe out sucking in the stomach as deep as you can. Continue this for 15 times.

Walk

Take a slow walk for about 30 minutes. Remember, the walk should be slow and lazily taken enjoying the scenario.

Sample Progress Chart

	Date	**1st Jan.**					
Spot Jogging	×	10 min.					
Jumping Jacks	×	20 min.					
Head rotation	×	5 min.					
Shoulder rotation	×	30 min.					
Knee rotation	×	30 min.					
Ankle rotation	×	30 times					
Side bends	×	20 times					
Front bends	×	5 times					
Lunges	×	5 times					
Back bends	×	3 times					

Contd...

	Date	1st Jan.					
Squats	×	20 times					
Dips	×	20 times					
Spot Jogging	×	20 times					
Jumping Jacks	×	50 times					
Sit-ups	×	20 times					
Leg raises	×	20 times					
Vacuum	×	15 times					
Walk	×	20 times					

The exercise duration and repetition has been given as an example for the first day of January. You can photocopy this chart and use it to fill in the detail of your workouts. After a week, you will find it easy and thus you can double everything and start jotting it down. At the end of the month, you will find that you can perform harder and longer.

Programme for Gaining Weight

Remember the idea here is not to gain weight in terms of fat. When I say 'gain weight' I mean gain muscular weight. And as we have already discussed, in order to gain muscular weight we need to eat right and rest and at the same time exercise appropriately.

If you are looking to gain muscular weight, I would suggest that you skip activities which result in excessive loss of calories. This means that activities like jogging, running, swimming; playing football, tennis and so on excessively are out of question. Here the idea is to conserve your calories; exercise in a way that the same calories are used up in building new muscle blocks.

Remember again, that rest is important. Only when you exercise and rest adequately will your muscles grow. If you maintain a hyperactive life, your calories will be used up and new muscular blocks will never be built.

Warm Up

Follow the same warm-up schedule as stated earlier in the Programme for Losing Weight section. The warm-up should be short and adequate. This means that with a short warm-up, your body should be adequately loosened up.

Training Programme

Follow the Joint Movements as stated earlier in the programme for Losing Weight. These movements prepare your body for the exercises coming up.

Squats

Squats should be done in a strict and rhythmic motion. Sit down bending your knees, but remember your hips should not touch your hamstring muscles (back portion of your thighs). Start by doing at least 30 repetitions. Within a week or two you should be able to increase your repetitions to at least a hundred in one go. A good idea here would be now to use some weights so that you could add some artificial resistance to your exercise, which will force your body to react into adjusting to the resistance, thereby gaining muscular weight.

You can use weight in various ways.

Hold a light dumb-bell on each of your hands as you squat. You can even put your palm on your lap resisting the straightening of the legs as you rise up. This puts added resistance to your exercise. However, I do not recommend using too much of weights doing these exercises.

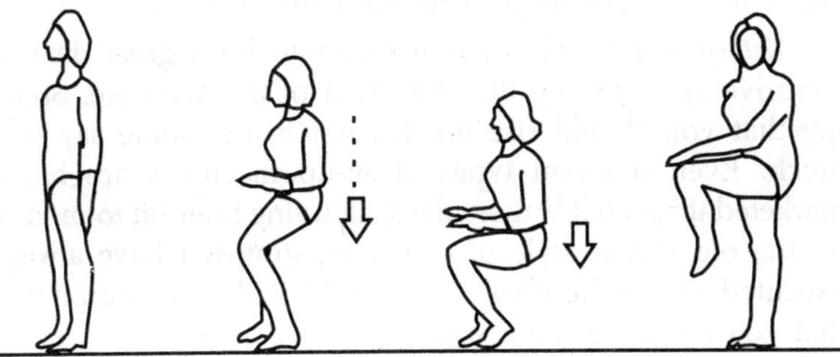

Dips

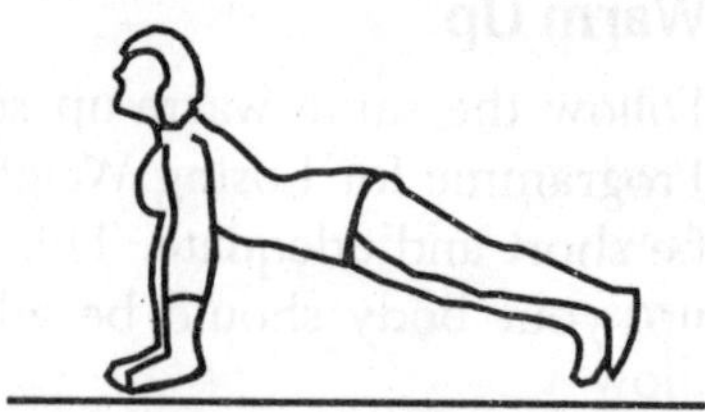

You can use dips to build the deltoids (shoulder muscles), pectorals (chest muscles), triceps and forearm flexor muscles by doing this exercise. Lie down facing the floor with your palms and the toe touching the floor. Raise your chest and upper body by straightening up your arms. Repeat this twenty times and increase the repetitions as you go on.

You can also add resistance while performing this exercise. There are various ways in which you can add resistance. One good idea would be to have a friend place a barbell plate on your back while you perform the exercise. If you have a kid brother or a sister, you can even provide a free ride for them on your back as you perform your exercise. This way, you will have a new fan and at the same time a good work-out. However, remember not to use too heavy a weight while performing this exercise if you are not used to handling weights.

Sit-Ups

You can use this exercise to build the upper abdominal muscles including the intercostal muscles. Repeat it 20 times and then increase the repetitions as you go on.

You can add resistance by having your friend place a barbell plate on your chest while you exercise. However, remember, if you are not used to working with weights you might find it very hard to perform this exercise.

Method of Execution: There seems to be a great deal of controversy regarding the execution of this exercise. Some say that you should rise up this much and some say that much. Even different types of sit-up machines are being marketed through TV these days, all trying their bit to modify on the old classic style of executing sit-ups. I have always executed sit-ups the classic way, and I will also recommend that you do it the same way.

Lie on your back, knees bent, feet flat on the floor, your hands on the outside of your thighs. Sit up and bring your head as close to your knees as possible. Lower yourself slowly back to the floor. After 20 reps you can use your arms to help you cheat a little by swinging them forward to allow you to do extra repetitions. Make sure you do this exercise very slowly and keep your chin pressed into your chest.

Variations: Working on the abs can only be optimally fruitful if you do a lot of variations. Hence include a lot of variations in your abs routine.

i) Twisting Sit-Ups

Twisting Sit-Ups is very good exercise to develop the upper abs while at the same time working on the intercostals. Here you involve the upper abs, external obliques as well as the intercostals, thus making it a complete upper abs exercise.

Method of Execution: Lie on your back, knees bent, feet flat on the floor, your hands behind your head. However, when you rise up, twist to bring your right elbow to your left knee and then, on the next repetition, your left elbow to your right knee, feeling each time a 'crunching' contraction of the intercostals.

Leg Raises

Leg Raises are predominantly lower abs exercise. You can use this exercise to define your lower abs.

Method of Execution: Sit up on the end of a flat bench (you may also do this lying down on the floor) and lie back with legs extended straight out and your hands underneath your buttocks

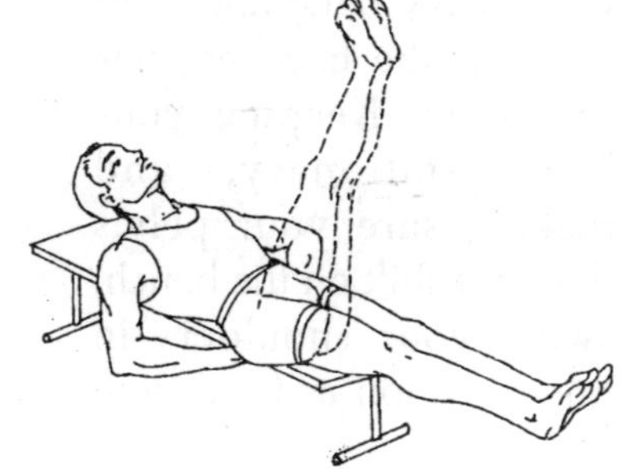

for support. Keeping your legs straight raise them as high as you can, then lower them slowly until they are below the level of the bench.

Remember for all Leg Raise movements it is important to tuck your chin forward into the chest in order to flex the upper abdominals during the exercise.

Bent-Knee Leg Raises

Bent-Knee Leg Raises also work the lower abs, however, they are much easier to execute than the former exercises.

Method of Execution: Start in the same position as the previous exercise. With your knees bent, raise them as high as possible toward your chest, then lower them slowly to the starting position.

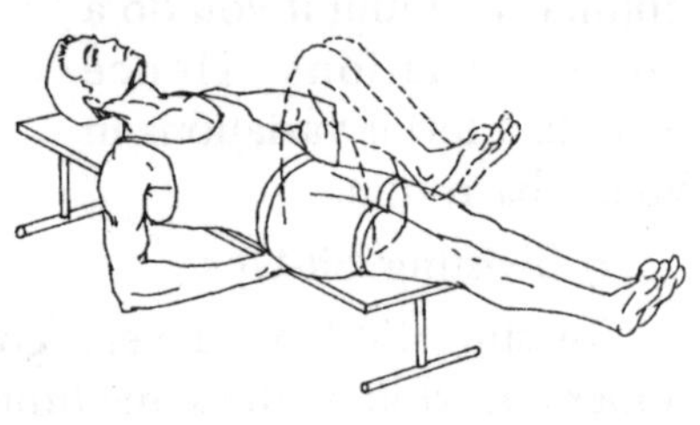

Seated Twists

This is one of my favourite exercises for working out the obliques resulting in that narrow waist which with the great sweep of the latissimus muscle complete the much wanted 'V' shape during the double biceps pose.

Method of Execution: Sit on the end of a bench, feet flat on the floor and comfortably apart. Take hold of a bar (don't use very heavy bars) and hold it across the back of your shoulders. Keeping your head stationary, and making sure your pelvis does not shift on the bench, swing your shoulders in one direction as far as you

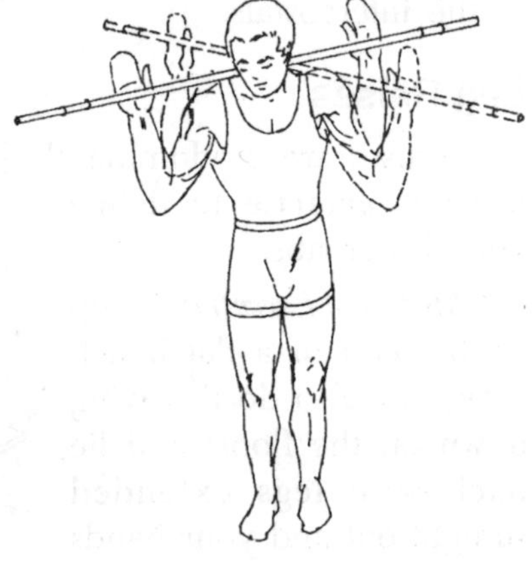

can, feeling the oblique muscles on that side fully contract. Come back to the centre then twist as far as you can in the other direction. As you get looser and more warmed up, increase the pace, swinging more energetically first in one direction, then reversing and swing back the other way.

Cool Down

As warm up is important, cool down is also important. It brings back the body temperature and circulation back to normal.

Vacuum (15 Times)

Stand upright. Take a deep breath and blow out your stomach as if it becomes a pumped balloon. Then breathe out sucking in the stomach as deep as you can. Continue this for 15 times.

Walk

Take a slow walk for about 20 minutes. Remember, the walk should be slow and lazily taken, enjoying the scenario.

OOO

For Working Men and Women

Computers could be a Health Hazard – how do you avoid it?

Are you a computer professional who has to work for hours end on at the computer? If yes, you could be slowly working towards the greatest health hazard of your life.

It is a known fact that for typists and those who are known to type a lot, whether working on the computer using a keyboard or the plain old typewriter, arthritis is a long forgone conclusion if not taken care of well in advance. The other factor about working on the computer starring at the 1024 x 768 pixels of electrons blasting at our retina every second is that it can lead to eye complications besides the daily stiff back and on the long term recurring back problems sitting on the chair. These are just the beginning of the never ending list of health complications that are bound to arise sooner or later for all serious computer users.

Now giving up using computers is surely not possible. However, a couple of smart and simple things can be followed in order to avoid all these computer oriented health hazards.

Here are some of the simple things that you might want to follow:

1. Never work on the computer for more than two hours at a stretch. If your work entails working on the computer for more than two hours continuously,

break up your work. For every two hours, give yourself a ten-minute break. Leave your terminal and come out under the sun to breathe some fresh air and stretch yourself. However, don't convert these breaks into 'cigarette breaks'.

2. Perform some of these exercises. Remember you can perform these exercises[1] right at your desk also.
   a. Wrist rotation[2] (both clockwise and anticlockwise).
   b. Open fingers and close one at a time with a squeezing motion. (You can even use a squeezing ball.)
   c. Bring your shoulders forward in a shrugging movement and return to the normal position[3]
   d. Raise your shoulders up and return to the normal position.
   e. Rotate your neck in both clockwise and anticlockwise movement
   f. Move your head to your left side and return to the normal position. Move your head now to your right side and return to the normal position.
   g. Sit up straight with your back firmly against the back of the chair. Hold this position for at least 15 seconds. Then lean forward towards your computer terminal and repeat the exercise again.
   h. Raise your legs, bending at the knee. Hold your knees close to the chest with your hands and maintain the position for 15 seconds. Return to the normal position.

---

[1] Each exercise can be performed for ten to fifteen repetitions, for each hand. The whole set can be repeated two to three times a day.

[2] These exercises are for the neck. Each exercise can be performed for 10-15 repetitions and the whole workout can be repeated twice or thrice a day. When doing these exercises, sit straight with your back firmly against the back of the chair. Arms should be close to the body and hands can rest on the thighs.

(Remember I am not suggesting that you perform all the exercises mentioned above. However, at least attempt some of them and work towards making a routine of sorts so that you do perform these exercises every day at work.)

3. While selecting a chair for working on the computer, be smart enough to select those chairs with good lower and mid-back support. Other specifications can be to your liking.

OOO

Men, Women and Job Stress

One of the leading causes of death recently among working men and women was stress related. Of course, a key component of the stress many men and women face in their jobs is the job itself. Work stress may increase the risk for cardiovascular disease, not to mention the detrimental psychological effect, workplace injury and/or other health problems. Managing work stress is thus not just of great importance but the only way to avoid these deadly afflictions.

We all tend to underestimate the threat of job stress. Most of the time we even label it to be a 'necessary evil'. And thus consequently, accept it as such. But is this truly the way it should be? I don't know but then again, stress is most definitely not a necessary evil.

In the United States, the respected Centers for Disease Control (CDC) describe work stress as, being *the harmful physical and emotional responses that occur when the requirements of a job do not match the capabilities, resources or needs of the worker. Early warning signs include headaches, sleep disturbances, difficulty concentrating, job dissatisfaction and low morale.*

When the body is under stress, the nervous system is aroused, hormones are released and as a result, we go into what is known as the 'fight or flight' response. Since most men and women would rather not run out of the office when this occurs, they normally opt for the 'fight' response. To many professionals, the word stress almost translates into the word 'challenge'. But of course, there is a difference.

Unlike stress, a challenge should energize and motivate an individual at the same time bringing with it a sense of satisfaction.

So, what do we do when anxiety and stress prevails? Sadly, many individual cope by turning to alcohol, drugs, food, sex, the TV remote control or prescription drugs for relief. However, there is another solution and a better one by far. And you probably know what is coming next - yes, exercise. Increasingly, it is becoming more common these days for professionals to use their lunch hour to hit for the gym. Doing so can relieve much stress as well as boost self-esteem and self-sufficiency. Both characteristics carry over into the work place.

Also instead of thinking of a workout as your exercise time, try to approach it as time you are taking for yourself to unwind; doing something just for you.

Surely there are two contrasts here - one is to use your exercise time to completely block out everything else in your daily grind while the other is to use the time to brainstorm. Many professionals say that they think of their best ideas or problem-solvers while doing simple exercises! Others say that time is a great escape for them. Whichever way works best for you is great. Some individuals of course, might not vouch for going to the gym. If this is you, take a walk instead. A simple 30-minute walk can do wonders for body and soul.

Whether we realize it or not, we all suffer from effects of stress. The next time you feel stressed out at work; do your best not to get angry. Give yourself the challenge of controlling your stress instead. Adopt a healthier lifestyle, even if only with a few minor changes such as a bit more activity and eating a bit healthier. Believe me, it all adds up!

OOO

De-stress within Minutes

Previously, we had discussed about the effects of stress at job. Now here are some simple steps which can help you to de-stress within minutes.

1. **Count:** Find a quiet and comfortable place to sit. Then take several slow, deep breaths to help clear your mind. Now continue breathing and repeating the word "one, two, three..." to yourself as you exhale. Practice this for two to three minutes once or twice a day. You should definitely find your stress levels dropping.
2. **Tune it out**: Known to ease out anxiety and lower blood pressure and heart rate, music is an old but tried and true stress buster. While slow music or soothing instruments typically yield the best results, choose a style you enjoy. Make it something that grabs you and takes your focus off your worries.
3. **Take a walk**: Any exercise, even a leisurely 30-minute walk or bike ride, can reduce stress. While you are exercising, do not let yourself think of anything that upsets you and causes stress. Rather, focus on what you are doing; the health benefits you are achieving. If you are taking a walk, look around at the scenery, if on a treadmill or stationery bike, put on some headphones with your favourite music. Whatever you do for your mind, do not let it worry!
4. **Write it out**: Put the details of a stressful event down on paper. This may help unburden your mind as well

as your body. Take 20 minutes a day, for three days and use that time to write about a stressful event in your life. Do not worry about spelling or style; just focus on getting it off your mind. When you are done with this, tear up your troubles and throw them out.

5. **Try an over-the-counter remedy:** Siberian ginseng is an herbal remedy available in health food stores and most pharmacies. It is great for bolstering the body against every day stress. Take 100mg in capsule form, three times a day for six months, followed by one dose a day for two months. Make sure the capsules standardize to one percentage *eleutherosides* to ensure you get enough of the active ingredient of the herb. Please note, however, if you are one who is sensitive to drugs and herbs, forget this suggestion or check with your doctor first.
6. **Customize your workspace**: One quick and easy way to ease workday tension is to make your desk or office feel more like home. Display snapshots of your last family vacation. Hang pictures or postcards of artwork or scenes you enjoy. Buy some fresh flowers and put them on your desk. These personal touches can help you relax even on your busiest day.

OOO

Play to remain Fit and Happy

Most professionals in their quest for career promotion forget that spending quality time with their kids is not simply what they owe to their kids, but most importantly, one of the most proven ways of de-stressing.

If you are married[1] and have kids, you can use the following playground favourites as your personal gym!

Swings

Pump your legs to swing higher using your quadriceps and hamstrings. The theory here is simple - The harder you pump, the higher you swing and the more intense your workout becomes. Now hop off and push your kid on the swing next. This will work your arms, or biceps. For an extra move that targets your abdominal muscles, you can sit on the swing; grasp the chains with your hands overhead while putting your kid at the same time on your lap.

The Slide

Climbing up the steps itself is good for your quadriceps, hamstrings and buttocks. The best part, however, is sliding down which does wonders for lifting your spirits and boosting your energy. If you are stuck at the bottom of the slide you

[1] And even if you aren't, taking your nieces, nephews or even the neighbour's kids wouldn't hurt.

can catch your child while she/he has all the fun and lift him/her overhead each time for a great upper-body workout.

Monkey Bars

Swinging from bar to bar alongside your kid is a fabulous workout for your upper body. So is climbing up and down the bars to exercise your arms and legs at the same time.

For an extra move that targets your arms, back and shoulders, you can do some chin-ups. If chin-ups are too difficult, do not sweat it, you can simply do these variations: Using a bar that is taller than you, place your hands about shoulder-width apart with your palms facing you. Step on a nearby bar to boost yourself up so your arms are bent and your chin is above the bar you are holding. Slowly lower your body by extending your arms. When your arms fully extend, use your feet to boost yourself back up.

Seesaw

The up-and-down motion is sure to put a smile on your face too, besides your kid's. And of course, the impact each time you land will help keep your bones strong, and pushing off to go back up works your legs and buttocks.

For an extra move that targets your chest, shoulders and arms, when it is not your turn to ride, use the main bar to do push-ups. Place your hands about shoulder-width apart and extend your legs behind you. Keeping your head back, and legs in a straight line, bend your elbows and slowly lower your chest toward the bar. Hold for a second then push back up.

There you have it. You had fun with your kids at the same time as you gave some time for yourself. There is no better way than this to look and feel younger as well as enjoy some quality time with your children! Imagine what fun it will be for them to see their parents enjoying with them at the playground also. Just think of the memories – and the great example you are setting by encouraging activity.

Here is the final tip:

To avoid accidents, always keep an eye on your kids, of course, and stick close by them. In fact, make this entire experience more fun for all by swinging with your kids and seesawing with them. If you have more than one child, set them both on the other end of the see-saw to challenge your leg muscles while you put them up into the air. If you do have to run after your child, or children, for any reason, that will burn calories as well. In addition, it will get your metabolism moving!

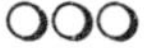

Soothe Tired Feet Instantly!

For how many times have you returned back home with your feet tired and heavy. Here is what you should do to soothe tired feet instantly.

Rub away fatigue and lower your risk of injury with a foot massage. Massaging the foot stimulates the nerve endings and rejuvenates the muscles. The better the shape you keep your feet in, the longer and stronger your walks will be and the lower your risk of injury. Please note, however, if you suffer from a contagious skin condition such as athlete's foot, or if you have diabetes, you should consult with your physician first.

Here's how you should massage your foot:

1. Work the sole of one clean, bare foot at a time. Start by moving the heel of your hand or thumb in long strokes from the heel to the base of the toes.
2. With a comfortable but firm pressure, use a fingertip or thumb to make little circles about the size of a 25 paise coin, all over the sole of the foot.
3. For deeper relief, press your thumb directly into one point on the sole and hold for a few seconds. Do this all over the bottom of your foot.
4. Grasping one toe at a time between your thumb and finger, simultaneously squeeze and tug gently along the length of the toe.

5. Finish by making little circles, as in step two, around the anklebones.

You can also do the following to soothe your feet:

1. Put a small but sturdy glass bottle or a cricket ball on the floor, and roll it under your foot, bearing down with a little pressure. If desired, chill the bottle for added relief.
2. Alternate hot and cold foot baths, soaking in hot water for five minutes, then cold water for 30 to 60 seconds.
3. Use specialty sandals or massage beds; both have nub insoles/bases to stimulate circulation.
4. Give yourself a special treat sometime when finances allow and splurge on a professional foot massage.

OOO

Sleep - The Basic Human Need

Sleep is a natural part of our life. But how many of us know how important it is?

Sleep is something our bodies need to do; it is not an option or something that we have a choice about. To sleep or not to sleep is thus not a question. Why, because sleep, like nutrition and exercise, is important for our minds and bodies to function normally. In fact, sleep is required for our very survival. Rats deprived of sleep die within two to three weeks, a time frame similar to death due to starvation.

According to scientific studies, an internal biological clock regulates the timing for sleep. It programmes each person to feel sleepy during the nighttime hours and to be active during the daylight hours. Light is thus the cue that synchronizes the biological clock to the 24-hour cycle of day and night.

Problem Sleepiness Has Serious Consequences

Sleepiness due to chronic lack of adequate sleep is a big problem in India and affects many children as well as adults. Children and even adolescents need at least 9 hours of sleep each night to do their best. Most adults need approximately 8 hours of sleep each night.

When we get less sleep (even one hour less) than we need each night, we develop a 'sleep debt.' If the sleep debt becomes too great, it can lead to problem sleepiness which is sleepiness that occurs when you should be awake and alert; this interferes with daily routine and activities, and reduces your ability to function. Even if you do not feel sleepy, the sleep debt can have a powerful negative effect on your daytime performance, thinking, and mood, and cause you to fall asleep at inappropriate and even dangerous times.

Problem sleepiness has other serious consequences as well. It puts adolescents and adults at risk for drowsy driving or workplace accidents. In children, it increases the risk of accidents and injuries. In addition, lack of sleep can have a negative effect on children's performance in school, on the playground, in extracurricular activities, and in social relationships.

Inadequate sleep can cause **decreases** in:

- Performance
- Concentration
- Reaction Times
- Consolidation of Information Learning

Inadequate sleep can also cause **increases** in:

- Memory Lapses
- Accidents and Injuries
- Behavioural Problems
- Mood Swings etc

Signs of Sleep Disorders

An individual who has not obtained adequate nighttime sleep is at high risk for symptoms of physical and/or mental impairment. He or she may fall asleep in the office, have difficulty concentrating in their work and other activities, and/or exhibit behavioural problems. Some individuals who are sleepy become agitated rather than lethargic and may be misdiagnosed as hyperactive. You should talk to your doctor about a possible sleep disorder if you have any of the following:

- Snoring
- Breathing Pauses During Sleep

- Problems with Sleeping at Night
- Difficulty Staying Awake During the Day
- Unexplained Decrease in Daytime Performance

Sleeping tips for all

If you are suffering from the inability to sleep, here are certain things that you might do before going to sleep.

1. Do not take a very heavy meal before going to sleep. If you do happen to take one, do not go to bed immediately. Instead, a short walk in the neighbourhood might do well.
2. While in bed make a habit of reading books, magazines or newspapers. However, do not indulge in smoking for nicotine has a tendency to keep you awake.
3. Never drink coffee or tea before going to bed. Alcohol also has the tendency to keep you awake.
4. While in bed, clear your mind of all thoughts and worries of either your work or your family. If you have a persisting problem say to yourself that you will sleep on it.
5. Do not think or contemplate while you are in the bed. These have a tendency to keep your mind agitated, leading to lack of concentration.
6. Maintain a routine of going to bed at around 9 pm. Avoid late night movies, parties or works.
7. And above all try to inculcate good and regular habits.

OOO

For Senior and Disabled Individuals

Exercise for Seniors

Research now indicates that men and women in their retirement years can do the same exercise routines as younger people and reap both physical and psychological benefits. However, the exercises should be performed at a slower pace to reduce any possibility of injury. One thing we cannot help is the fact that as we age, we are more susceptible to injury - no matter how much of a great shape we are in.

If you are elderly and healthy, all you need do is continue working hard, as much as you feel you can. You should not overdo it however, but do enough that you feel you are working at a challenging pace. This way, you will definitely see results.

Free hand exercises, including aerobic movements, are the most highly recommended way to build strength and stamina, not only for the elderly but for those of all ages. You get a mental boost as well as physical improvements. In addition, those who work out regularly fall less and consequently, suffer fewer injuries. Currently, falling is the leading cause of all injury-related deaths among India's senior citizens.

OOO

Exercise Tips for Seniors

Before we begin, please note that if you have a family history of heart disease, check with your doctor first. It is a good idea to have a physical examination before you start any exercise programme. However, if you are healthy and your doctor gives you the go ahead, then pick rhythmic, repetitive activities that challenge the circulatory system and exercise at an intensity appropriate for you.

Choose activities that are fun, suit your needs and that you can do year-round.

Wear comfortable clothing and footwear appropriate for the temperature, humidity and activity.

If you decide that walking is a great activity for you, choose a place that has a smooth, soft surface and does not intersect with traffic and is well lighted and safe. This is why many senior Indians walk in the parks.

Find a companion to exercise with you, if it will help you stay on a regular schedule and add to your enjoyment.

Because muscular adaptation and elasticity generally slows with age, take more time to warm up and cool down while exercising. Also make sure you stretch slowly. Start exercising at a low intensity, especially if you have been mostly sedentary, and progress gradually.

If you plan to be active more than 30 minutes, then try to drink some water every 15 minutes, especially when exercising in hot, humid conditions. As you age, your sense of thirst tends to decrease and you cannot completely rely on your internal sense of thirst.

OOO

Walking our way to a Healthy Life

"Just doing thirty minutes of walking, five times a week, can reduce your risk of developing diabetes by as much as 58 per cent," says Centers for Disease Control (CDC)[1] in its recent study.

Indeed to improve your health, all you need to do is walk. Walking is a great way to accustom your body to exercise. Thirty minutes of brisk walking has been proved to reduce the risk of cardiovascular disease by as much as 40 per cent. Cardiovascular disease is the number one killer of both men and women in India today.

Of course, for many of you, walking may not seem like much of an exercise, but it can surely make a world of difference. It can lift your spirits. It can definitely make you feel more at ease. You can feel a sense of accomplishment. And all of these, just by getting out and walking.

Depression and Walking

Walking can also be part of managing depression. A quick walk every day makes you feel more positive and more in control. Walking releases *endorphins*, the anti-stress, feel-good hormones naturally produced by your body. Research shows

[1] CDC is one of the most respected Government Agencies in the United States

that *endorphins* are natural 'mood elevators'. They are responsible for the 'runner's high' feeling you get after being active.

Walking also relieves stress, a common side effect of depression. So, just breaking your routine with a simple walk can help both body and mind feel better.

You will find walking can help you in other ways, too. You will burn more calories. This can help you stay in shape and keep you looking good. When you look good, you feel better and have more confidence in yourself.

Some tips

Of course, I need not tell you how to walk, but certainly there are things that you might want to do before going for a walk.

1. It would be a good idea to properly dress first. If it is cold, cover yourself up well. And if it is warm, cover yourself just as well-being smart to wear clothes which offer good internal air circulation.
2. Always carry a small napkin to wipe your perspiration.
3. Wear runners that are comfortable and well ventilated. It must have a good internal air circulation.
4. If you have partners, don't talk too much while you walk. This will lead to breathlessness and you will have to rest or get back your breath every now and then.
5. If you like to keep walking distance targets, do keep realistic targets. Don't say, "Today, I will walk 5 km." You might not make it and this might lead to self-disappointment.
6. Above all, enjoy your walk. Don't think of it as a challenge of sorts or something that you do to prove yourself. Think of it instead as something that you love and have a lot of fun doing it.

OOO

Meditation for Seniors

Elderly people who practice meditation can drastically reduce their medical costs, according to findings presented by Robert Herron at the 91st Annual Canadian Public Health Association Conference in 2003 in Ottawa, Canada[1].

Dr. Herron's study found that 163 people from Quebec - aged 65 and over - reduced payments to physicians by a cumulative 70 per cent during the five-year period after they learned Meditation.

The retrospective study evaluated a sample of 326 Quebec health insurance enrollees - 163 who practiced Meditation technique and 163 who did not. Using statistical analysis, researchers compared the groups' expenses for treatment by physicians, both during the nine-year period before Meditation was introduced and for five years afterward. Data for the study was provided by the *Regie de l'Assurance-Maladie du Quebec*, the province's health insurance provider. Figures were adjusted for inflation using the Canadian government's Consumer Price Index.

The study's findings were dramatic. Researchers found 70 per cent cumulative expenditure reduction for the group who practiced Meditation technique for five years. In contrast, the control group's expenses continued to rise. Both groups

---

1 Herron RE, Cavanaugh K.; 2001; "Can Meditation Reduce Medical Expenditures of Older People?" In the *Journal of Social Behaviour and Personality.*

showed steadily rising payments to physicians during the nine-year period before the group learned Meditation.

"These findings suggest that there is a relationship between Meditation and improved mental and physical health for senior citizens," said Dr. Herron, lead author of the study. "The proven health benefits of meditation could have significant implications for the reduction of medical costs for people of all ages."

OOO

Protect Yourself against Health Fraud

Indians spend crores of rupees each year on products or services that claim everything from "losing weight while you sleep" to "no more arthritic pain." Easy remedies are hard to resist, but many don't always deliver on their promises. Some can even be harmful.

Health-fraud means promoting, for financial gain, a health remedy that doesn't work or simply hasn't yet been proven to work. Health-fraud has grown significantly in the past several years. Why? Because people today take more personal responsibility for staying healthy. And this interest has launched a huge demand for products and services that promote health.

What are the consequences? Well, health fraud takes advantage of consumers and involves significant economic and health risks, including:

False Hopes

Unsound nutrition advice, products or services won't prevent or cure disease. For the best advice, you must always contact your physician and a dietetics professional such as a registered dietitian.

A Substitute for Reliable Health Care

Remember proper health care can be delayed if you follow bad advice. You may lose something you can't retrieve, for example, time for an effective treatment.

Unneeded Expense

Even under the best of circumstances, some products and services simply don't work. Why should you then waste your hard-earned money on something that has no effect?

Potential Harm

Unsound nutrition advice, products or services can put your health at risk. Large doses of some vitamins and minerals, in the form of dietary supplements, can have harmful side effects. For example, excessive vitamin K is risky if you take blood-thinning drugs.

What can you do to protect yourself from such fraudulent activities?

Simply follow these tips:

Always do Your Homework

Find out more before you purchase a nutrition product, treatment or service.

Seek Advice from Reliable Sources

It's not easy to distinguish facts from misinformation. Contact a credible source such as your doctor for advice.

Report Such Frauds

If you suspect that a statement, product or service is false, discuss it with the appropriate government agency or file a complaint at a nearby police station.

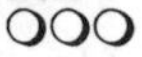

Working Out Safely with High Blood Pressure

The fllowing are some simple and safe tips for improving the health of your heart. Regular aerobic exercise can lower both systolic and diastolic blood pressure by an average of ten points. However, because exercise does make your heart work harder, you need to be careful, especially if you are just starting an exercise regime or if your blood pressure is excessively high. (Greater than 159/99)

To exercise safely, follow these tips:

Be Moderate

Avoid competitive exercises that include bursts of intense exertion. Easy aerobic exercise such as walking is good for people of all blood pressure levels.

Stand Slowly

After stretching or exercising on the floor, get up slowly. Some blood pressure medications can cause "orthostatic hypotension", a condition that makes you dizzy when you stand quickly.

Do it Daily

Consistent exercise lowers blood pressure best. Try to work out at least four days a week, daily if possible. For best results, try doing at least 20 minutes each time.

Skip Caffeine

A pre-workout cup of coffee may cause a spike in blood pressure. Avoid caffeine three to four hours before exercising.

Warm-up and Cool down

Always warm-up and cool down to help your body heat adjust to activity.

OOO

Training Your Memory

Surely you must have heard the expression, 'Use it or lose it'. Believe me, this can apply to our memories as well. One of the most common fears among seniors is the loss of memory and what it could mean to their health, well-being and relationships. Statistics show 80 per cent of seniors are concerned about their memory on a daily basis. If this is you, you are not alone and this concern is not something you should take lightly at any stage of life. You can take some control of your own destiny by constantly self-educating.

Here are some important means by which you could remain mentally fit:

1. Older adults can improve their memory or retain their memory by simply challenging their minds with puzzles, reading, trivia games and a computer. Staying interested in things and learning all you can about them are important throughout our entire lives. One could take up a hobby that requires concentration and following directions. There are many things we can do to retain our mental capabilities. Find ways to amuse and entertain yourself and if you are able, stay as active socially as possible.
2. It is true that coffee gives seniors a memory boost. If you are over the age of 65, a cup of java can jog your memory. Studies show that memory in senior citizens is best in the morning but wanes as the day goes on. By about 4 p.m. a cup of coffee may be just the ticket

to tune up your memory for the remainder of the day. This is not an official endorsement of coffee though, but the results are irrefutable.

3. Mediate at least 15 to 20 minutes a day.
4. Sleep well and eat lots of green vegetables. A small meal at around 4 pm consisting of a lot of green vegetables tunes up the spirits of the seniors.
5. You should eat small but frequent meals. And above all drink a lot of water.

OOO

Diet and Nutrition

Eating Your Way to Good Health

The Ten Commandments of Dieting

1. Aim for a healthy weight. You can give yourself a quick check to see if you should weigh in less with a tape measure. Measure around the smallest part of your waist. Women shouldn't exceed a 35-inch waist. Men shouldn't exceed a 40-inch waist.
2. Be physically active each day. Adults should try to get about 30 minutes of moderate exercise each day and children can use a full hour.
3. Do your best to choose your foods from the food pyramid. Here are the guidelines:
   - Nine servings of bread, cereal or noodles
   - Four servings of vegetables
   - Three servings of fruit
   - Two or three servings of dairy
   - Two servings of meat, fish or poultry

   This sounds like a lot, but serving sizes are a lot smaller than one realizes. We've become a society of a large everything, distorting our impression of an average serving size.

   Here are some ways to determine a proper portion size without having to weigh or measure:

1 cup: The size of your fist.

Example: About two servings of oatmeal.

1 ounce: The size of your entire thumb.

Example: A piece of cheese

1 or 2 ounces of a snack food: A handful.

Example: 1 ounce nuts=1 handful equals 2 ounces; pretzels=2 handfuls.

Single serving of margarine: Thumb tip

Example: A small dip of the knife (do not make it a huge dip!)

3 ounces: Palm of your hand

Example: A cooked serving of meat

4. Eat a variety of grains every day. This amount equals six to nine servings, three of which should be whole grains.
5. Keep foods safe to eat. Observe proper refrigeration and adequate cooking temperatures.
6. Adhere to a diet low in saturated fat and cholesterol.
7. Reduce your intake of soft drinks containing sugar.
8. Cut down on salt. Use herbs and seasonings instead.
9. Avoid alcohol.
10. Accept the fact that there is no easy quick fix for losing weight. Eating less and exercising more are the keys to successful weight loss and optimal health.

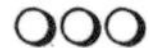

Are you getting enough of Fruits and Vegetables?

Indians fall very short of the goal to eat five servings of vegetables and four servings of fruit. These guidelines are daunting at best. When one is dieting or watching the scale, this sounds like a perfect formula that would blow all your dieting triumphs, forcing you to choose between being overweight or healthy! I think, however, the following information may be helpful to help sum this up into an eating plan that makes more sense for all.

One fruit serving consists of:

• 1 small to medium piece of fruit • 1 cup raw (cutup) fruit • ½ cup (4 ounces) fruit juice • ¼ cup dried fruit ½ cup canned fruit • ½ of a banana

One serving of vegetables consists of:

• ½ cup cooked vegetables • 1 cup raw, leafy vegetables • ½ cup (4 ounces) vegetable juice

To achieve these dietary goals, it is a good idea to take a proactive approach. With a very small investment of time, you and your family can eat nutritious meals that include an abundance of fruits and vegetables. When you go to a grocery shopping, try to account for five to nine servings of produce per day per family member.

To incorporate this into your daily diet, try to get the day off to a good start by eating two servings of fruit at breakfast time. This could be a banana sliced into a bowl of cereal, already accounting for two servings, or a fruit smoothie made with skim milk and one to two cups fresh or frozen berries. Choose whole fruit over juice to boost overall fibre content for the day. In general, limit fruit juice to one cup a day for two of your fruit servings.

When packing lunches and snacks, try to include two fruit and two vegetable servings. Even if you typically go out for lunch, this is still a good habit. You will then have these items available to snack on throughout the day. A low-sodium tomato juice and one cup of raw fresh vegetables would cover the vegetable requirement. For fruit, add a cup of grapes and a nectarine or a pear. Use pre-cut, bagged salad mixes you simply rinse, toss and serve. When choosing a salad mix, darker green means more nutrients. Add fruits such as apples, pears or dried cranberries to salads.

If you are not serving a salad, include cooked fresh or frozen vegetables for dinner. Your dinner plate should be half full of cooked vegetables to ensure three servings of vegetables for dinner. If you often eat out, make an effort to include a salad or cooked vegetable in your selection.

Are you still feeling overwhelmed? It can sound like a bit too much, even with this attempt to simplify the problem. To prevent boredom, choose a variety of textures and colors and do not be afraid to try something new. Here is a sample meal providing four fruit and five vegetable servings in a day.

BREAKFAST: Two fruits
SNACK: One fruit
LUNCH: Two vegetables and one fruit
SUPPER: Three vegetables

Whether you are cooking at home, eating at a restaurant at work or on the road a lot, it is still possible for you to get your daily requirement of fruits and vegetables. A little planning and ingenuity can go a long way!

OOO

Protein vs. Carbohydrates: A Weight-Loss Choice?

With more and more of Indians overweight or obese, the experts are debating what kinds of foods put on the weight. A balanced diet is the best way to prevent cancer and heart disease while managing your weight.

But what is making Indians overweight - the fat or the carbohydrates? People all across the country are debating this issue. Do you lose weight by eliminating most of the fat in your diet? Or do you shed those kilos by eliminating the carbohydrates and filling up on protein along with the saturated fat that comes with it?

Neither of course! If you want to lose weight and stay healthy, you have to eat fewer calories and exercise more, not simply cut whole categories of foods from your diet.

The stakes in this debate are high because certain kinds of fat are linked to higher long-term risk for cancer and other chronic diseases. On the other hand, certain types of carbohydrates - particularly vegetables and fruit - are linked to lowering that risk.

Choosing Healthful Fats and Carbohydrates

Originally, health experts recommended reducing overall fat intake for heart health and lower weight. However, recent research shows that some fats, used in moderation, may have health benefits. Highly monounsaturated fats like olive and canola oil are considered to be 'heart healthy.' Similarly, laboratory tests suggest that omega-3 fatty acids (found in fatty fish, flaxseed, walnuts, and canola and soybean oils) may help protect against cancer.

The questionable fats that some cancer research studies show to be hazardous are saturated fats from animal proteins, such as red meat, whole milk and butter. Health experts also advise avoiding products using 'partially hydrogenated vegetable oil,' which contain harmful trans-fatty acids. Most margarine also contains trans-fats, but after public protests, some companies have manufactured versions without trans-fets; so just check the labels when you buy one.

At the same time, some scientists argue that refined carbohydrates like white sugar, white rice and processed cereals raise insulin levels. In turn, this leads to overeating and storage of excess fat at the waist and hips. So they recommend unrefined carbohydrates such as whole wheat, brown rice and bran cereals which are digested more slowly and contain dietary fibre that solid research evidence shows is linked to lower colon cancer risk.

The cancer-fighting vitamins and phytochemicals in fibre-rich vegetables, fruits, whole grains and beans are another important health benefit. Dismissing these foods simply because they are carbohydrates is short-sighted.

Abandoning fruits and vegetables because they also contain carbohydrates could prove disastrous to your health. A much wiser course is to eat moderate portions of the types of carbohydrates and fats that are good for long-term health.

Eat Less and Exercise More for Weight Loss

For those concerned about weight loss, reducing portion size and increasing physical activity level is the best course. Experts believe that promotional practices such as 'supersizing' and 'value marketing' have confused people about reasonable portion sizes. As a result they are consuming approximately 148 more calories per day than they were two decades ago. These added calories could amount to a weight gain of 15 pounds per year.

As you compose your meals to be 2/3 plant-based foods and 1/3 animal protein, gradually reduce the size of portions. Ask yourself how many of those standard serving sizes go into the portions you usually eat, and use them as a guide to adjust your diet to be more healthful. Reduce your portion sizes gradually. Then add more physical activity to your schedule, and weight loss will probably result.

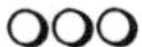

Ten Ways to Good Nutrition

1. The major dietary problem in India and most of the other developing countries is over-consumption of certain dietary components. Excessive intake of sugars and fats has resulted in excessive caloric intake together with a diet of low nutrient density.
2. The evidence that diets restricted in fat, saturated fat and cholesterol can reduce the incidence of chronic diseases is now overwhelming.
3. Learn to recognize the difference between hunger and appetite. Hunger is the stimulus within our bodies that indicates to us that we need to consume food. Appetite consists of the pleasurable sensations provided by food and is associated with the enjoyment of food.
4. Food is often used in one way or another to express feelings of happiness, love, security, or to cover up emotions of worry, grief, and loneliness and so on. Before you have a snack, ask yourself why you need this snack, or why you may be reaching for something you know you should not eat.
5. There is a saying, "A healthy body produces a healthy mind." This is true, because the brain benefits when food intake is adequate.
6. Support of family and friends is necessary for success.
7. Whatever you eat turns into you. Only you have complete control of what goes into your mouth.

8. Sugar. Be careful. It is very easy to eat excess amounts of sugary food which raise to a very high level your caloric intake.
9. An important part of staying fit is controlling your body weight.
10. Food is anything that nourishes the body. No two foods are alike in the ability to nourish, for no two foods contain identical amounts of nutrients. Therefore, variety in your diet is important.

OOO

Frequently Asked Questions

Aerobics

What is an Aerobic Exercise?

Answer: The word "aerobic" literally means "with oxygen" or "in the presence of oxygen." Aerobic exercise is any activity that uses large muscle groups, can be maintained continuously for a long period of time and is rhythmic in nature. Aerobic activity stimulates the heart, lungs and cardiovascular system to process and deliver oxygen more quickly and efficiently to every part of the body. As the heart muscle becomes stronger and more efficient, a larger amount of blood can be pumped with each stroke. Fewer strokes are then required to rapidly transport oxygen to all parts of the body. An aerobically fit individual can work longer, more vigorously and achieve a quicker recovery at the end of the aerobic session.

What Factors Affect Aerobic Training?

Answer: Frequency, duration and intensity. Frequency refers to how often you perform aerobic activity, duration refers to the time spent at each session, and intensity refers to the percentage of your maximum heart rate or heart rate reserve at which you work.

How do I Determine My Target Heart Rate?

Answer: The general formula for the average person is 220–age times 60% and times 90% of HRmax. For example, a 30-year old would calculate his target zone using the above formula: 220–30 = 190. 190 × .60 = 114 and 190 × .90 = 171. This individual would try to keep his heart rate between 114 (low end) and 171 (high end) beats per minute.

The Karvonen Formula calculates your heart rate reserve range. To calculate it, take your pulse for one minute on three successive mornings upon waking up. (We will be using the case of a 30-year old male whose resting pulse was 69, 70 and 71 for an average of 70 over the 3 days.)

Calculate target heart rate by subtracting your age from 220 (220–30 = 190).

Subtract your average resting heart rate from target heart rate (190–70 = 120).

The lower boundary of the percentage range is 50% of this plus your resting heart rate [(120 × .5) + 70 = 130]. The higher boundary is 85% plus your RHR [(120 × .85) + 70 = 178]. Using the Karvonen Formula for percentage of heart rate reserve, this 30-year old man should be working between 130 and 178 BPM.

Like the maximum heart rate formula, the Karvonen formula can vary from individual to individual. Not every individual is "average", and there can be large differences among people. Therefore, heart rate alone may not be the best indicator of how hard or how well you are working.

It is important to note that the deviation in both the age-specific formula and the Karvonen formula is due to the estimation of HRmax (Maximum heart rate). If you have an actual HRmax from a graded exercise test, it will be more accurate. ACSM lists two formulas for estimating HRmax, each one with a standard deviation of +/– 10-12 BPM:

HRmax = 220 – age (low estimate) HRmax

= 210 – (0.5 × age) (high estimate)

HR = Exercise intensity × HRmax × 1.15

Source: ACSM's Guidelines for Exercise Testing and Prescription, 5th Edition, p. 274, Williams and Wilkins.

What are Some Other Methods for Determining My Workout Intensity?

Answer: The Borg scale of perceived exertion is another way of determining how hard you are working. Using your own subjective Rate of Perceived Exertion (RPE) on a scale of 6-20 or a scale of zero-10, you determine how hard you are working. A rating of 12-16 ("somewhat hard" to "hard" on the 12-20 scale) or a rating of 4-6 ("somewhat strong" to "very strong") on the 0-10 scale reflects a heart rate of 60-90% of maximum and should be the target area for which to strive.

Original Scale		Revised Scale	
6		0	Nothing at all
7	Very, very light	0.5	Very, very weak
8		1	Very weak
9	Very light	2	Weak
10		3	Moderate
11	Fairly light	4	Somewhat strong
12		5	Strong
13	Somewhat hard	6	
14		7	Very strong
15	Hard	8	
16		9	
17	Very hard	10	Very, very strong
18		*	Maximal
19	Very, very hard		
20			

Source: ACSM's Guidelines for Exercise Testing and Prescription, 5th Edition, p. 68, Williams and Wilkins

The talk test is another measure of intensity. You should be able to talk without gasping for air while working at optimal intensity. If you cannot, you should scale down.

I do Lots of Outer Thigh (Tummy, Buns, etc.). Will That Part of My Body Slim Down First?

Answer: No. When we're working a muscle or group of muscles to burn fat, we have no control over what part of the body we burn fat from. There is no such thing as "spot reducing". Fat generally is used up in pretty much the reverse order it was put on, (LIFO–Last In First Out). When you are exercising, the blood is carrying fat from all over the body to provide the energy. The muscles which are being worked upon, will improve, of course, so when the layers of fat finally do get worked off, you'll have some nice lean tissue to show for all your efforts.

Another aspect to this question is the fact that muscle growth underneath a fat deposit can give the appearance of spot reduction. This is because the overlying fat is stretched over a greater surface and appears thinner, although the total amount of fat is the same. A good analogy is that of a balloon. As the air is increased, the skin on the balloon gets thinner, but the amount of balloon material stays the same. I think that this may be how the spot reduction myth originated. By working the muscles below the fat, people think they are actually making the fat go away.

How do I Know When I'm Exercising Hard Enough to Burn Fat?

Answer: Actually, you're almost always burning fat at one rate or another, but you burn most when your body is in its aerobic range. A good rule of thumb is that after 20 minutes in your aerobic zone, you will be burning more fat than carbos. Covert Bailey, in *Smart Exercise,* states that you will be burning fat after only twelve minutes of aerobic exercise. If you can increase your aerobic activity to 30 minutes or longer, you will be burning a larger percentage of calories from fat. There is still some disagreement as to which is better–longer duration at lower intensity, or shorter duration at higher intensity. If you are limited by time, then the higher intensity will maximize your aerobic benefits in a shorter amount of time. If you can work for a longer duration at a lower intensity, you will decrease your chance of injury. The aim is to burn more calories than you take in. 3,500 calories equal l pound of fat. Your muscles will continue to burn fat after both aerobic and anaerobic (muscle training) exercise.

This is perhaps the most common question raised by individuals exercising for the purpose of either weight loss or simply weight control. This stems from the recognition that aerobic exercise is a significant adjunct to any weight loss programme, that is, diet plus aerobic exercise produces more weight loss than diet alone. In addition, the weight lost with exercise tends to be a higher percentage of fat.

Exercise can be grouped into three broad levels of intensity–mild, moderate and high. Mild intensity is a comfortable walking pace and can be sustained almost indefinitely. Moderate intensity is equal to an average cardiovascular conditioning workout (able to talk, but not sing) and can be sustained (in a trained individual) for 3-4 hours, and high intensity is not able to talk and can only be sustained for 30-45 minutes.

Based on recent and very detailed research studies, in terms of absolute fat burning, a moderate intensity workout burns much fat. At a heart rate equal to about 75% of max, fat burning will approach 0.5 grams-1.0 grams of fat per minute. There is a weight dependence with the lower end referring to a 100–pound individual and the upper end to a 200–pound person. As the duration continues (greater than 1 hour), fat burning can increase slightly (another 10%).

At a mild intensity, the majority of calories expended (85-90%) are fat calories, but the absolute level is only about 60% of the moderate intensity. At high intensity levels, fat burning declines to a level of about 65% of the moderate pace, as sugar burning supplies the rest. The high rate of sugar burning exhausts the limited sugar supply in muscles and causes muscular failure.

The only caveats for the above burn rates are that these numbers are derived from individuals who were already aerobically trained and were conducted before breakfast. Less fit individuals are known to burn less fat and more sugar (part of aerobic conditioning is greater reliance on fat burning for energy). Exercising after a meal will tend to promote more sugar burning. Consumption of sugar during an exercise session will also tend to retard fat burning in favour of the sugar. These numbers were derived from cycling and so the absolute numbers can be increased if exercises that involve more muscle groups are utilized (running, rowing, etc.). From peak energy production rates for various exercises, rowers might reach about 40% higher.

Is It Better to Break My Exercise Sessions, or Exercise for a Longer Period?

Answer: There are two distinct thoughts on this issue; both present fairly reasonable arguments.

1. First, it takes 15-20 minutes to get your metabolism into the fat burning zone that many people desire for an aerobic workout. Once you have reached this level, your body tends to obtain more of its energy from fat than carbohydrates. Using this argument, a single 90-minute workout will allow you to exercise in this "fat burning" zone for at least 70 minutes while two 45-minute sessions would allow you to be in this zone for at least 50 minutes (2×25). This logic supports a single, longer workout.
2. Second, for about 6 hours after a workout, your body remains in "after burn" mode, burning more calories at rest than it would have if you had not worked out. Using this logic, two sessions would produce two after burn periods and result in more fat being burned than would be possible by a single workout session.

The real bottom line is that if you exercise for 90 minutes a day, you're interested in more than just fitness. To stay in reasonable cardiovascular shape, you need to perform aerobically for 20-30 minutes at least 3 times a week. If you wish to be in better than "the minimum acceptable" shape, remember that the returns are not geometric (you won't be in twice as good shape if you work out for twice as long). Therefore, if you're going to work out for 90 minutes a day, splitting the time between one or two sessions probably doesn't make a significant fitness-level difference.

How Much Should I Weigh?

Answer: What you weigh is not as important as the percentage of body fat to lean tissue. You can be overweight without being overfat and vice versa. Since muscle weighs more per volume than fat, and you want to have firm muscles throughout your body, you may weigh more than you thought was average for your height and build. There is still much controversy over what is "ideal" bodyweight. While some body fat is essential to sustain life, it is generally thought that a healthy body fat percentage for males is 8-20% and for females is 13-25%.

What's the Best Way to Determine Body Fat Percentage?

Answer: Weighing in water (hydrostatic) is generally considered the best method. But, the real answer is that a single measurement, no matter how accurate, doesn't tell you much. What's really important is, are you gaining or losing fat? The best way to answer this question is to take a reading every few weeks and graph the results. The absolute accuracy of these readings isn't really important as long as you use consistent technique so that the error is about the same every time.

The two methods that work best for at-home measurements are skin-fold calipers and biceps IR units. Treat the numbers not as "body fat percentage" but as a "body fat index." If, after several readings, your body fat index is clearly trending up, you may want to reconsider your diet and exercise programmes. It's like the petrol gauge in your car– it doesn't tell you how many litres you have, but it gives you a relative indication.

Should I Train My Muscles As Well As do Aerobic Activity?

Answer: Definitely. Muscle training is an integral part of any aerobic programme. After muscle training, our bodies continue to burn fat for many hours. The combination of aerobic exercise, muscle training, proper diet and stretching is an excellent programme for getting fit and staying healthy.

Which is Better for Muscle Training– Weights or Exertubes (Dynabands)?

Answer: Neither is actually "better". All exercise accessories have their uses. Weights require more muscles in use to maintain proper form, while the bands and tubes are easier to use in targeting specific muscles. Bands and tubes also have the advantage of being somewhat adjustable in resistance just by changing length. To change weights in dumb-bells, you either need another set of dumb-bells, or extra plates for those which use plates. Dumb-bells, however, do offer a much greater range of available weights, particularly at the high end, making them more useful in strength training. Bands and tubes are generally used in resistance training exercises.

What is a Cool Down and How Important is it to the Aerobic Activity?

Answer: After any aerobic activity, the blood is pooled in the extremities, and the heart rate is elevated. The purpose of the cooldown is to bring the heart rate down to near-normal and to get the blood circulating freely back to the heart. Stopping abruptly could result in fainting or place undue stress on the heart. The cooldown should also include stretching to help relax the muscles which worked so hard during the activity. The cool-down stretches also increase flexibility, and might help to prevent DOMS (Delayed Onset Muscle Soreness), although this has not been proven.

Should I Use Steam, a Sauna, or a Hot Tub Right After a Workout?

Answer: Since the blood tends to pool in your extremities after a vigorous workout, and steams, saunas, hot tubs and even hot showers tend to dilate your blood vessels, it is really not the best thing to do as it will be more difficult for the blood to reach the heart and brain. However, if you've done a thorough aerobic cooldown, and you wait for a reasonable amount of time to return to almost normal, you might go into one of these "fun" things. But if you feel any sign of weakness or dizziness, get out immediately.

I Never Exercised Before. How should I Begin?

Answer: It is a good idea to start slowly and build up to a full programme. Walking is the easiest way to begin a programme. Start with a stroll for a kilometre or so and build up to walking 3-4 kilometres per hour. As you become proficient at walking, you might want to try another activity such as jogging, running or even aerobic or step classes. The best aerobic programme is the one you enjoy and will stick to. Remember, the journey of a thousand kilometres begins with but a single step.

What is Step Aerobics?

Answer: Step aerobics is a form of aerobic activity which is performed on a platform that usually ranges from 4" to 10" in height. Step training was developed to provide a low-impact activity that is both challenging and interesting. People, who may not like certain aspects of aerobic dance, find that step is a very good alternative. Each participant works within his or her own space. There is no traveling across a room. When done properly, step training is an efficient means of improving aerobic fitness.

What are the Proper Stepping Techniques?

Answer: Your body should remain in good alignment. Your head should be up, shoulders down and back, chest up, abdominals and buttocks tight. When stepping up, lean from the ankles and not the waist to avoid placing excessive stress on the lumber spine. Contact the platform with the entire foot. To avoid Achilles tendon injury, make sure your heel is down, and your foot is in the centre of the platform. When stepping down, step close to the platform and allow the heels to contact the floor to help absorb the shock. (toe, ball, heel). When doing lunges or repeater steps, however, the heel should be up, and the weight should be on the forefoot of the working leg. You should not use hand or leg weights when you are stepping as the risk of injury outweighs any added benefit you might get from using weights. It is important to note, that anyone with a history of knee problems should consult a physician before beginning step training.

How High should My Step be?

Answer: Step height depends on several things– fitness level, current stepping skill, and the degree of knee flexion when the knee is fully loaded while stepping up. At no time should the knee joint of the first leg to step up flex beyond a 90° angle. Reebok is now saying that 60° is even better. De-conditioned individuals or beginners should begin on a 4" platform. As you improve, you may add risers to increase the step height making sure not to exceed the 90° of knee flexion. The most popular step heights are 6" and 8".

How can I Increase My Intensity?

Answer: There are several ways to increase intensity. Increase your step height, use longer lever arms or add propulsion moves (where both feet are off the step at the same time). If you are going to add propulsion, or power as it is known today, make sure not to do these moves for more than one minute at a time as these moves result in higher vertical impact. All power moves should be done as you go up onto the platform. Always step down without power. Power moves are considered advanced, and should not be attempted by beginners.

How Fast should the Music be?

Answer: According to Step Reebok guidelines, music should be played at a speed of 118-122 BPM. Technique and safety are seriously compromised when the music is too fast. It is also impossible to get the full range of motion that can be achieved at slower tempos.

Exercise and Eating

How Long should I Wait for Exercise After Eating?

Answer: If you ate something fairly light, you probably don't need to wait for very long. However, since people are different, it is difficult to say what the optimum waiting period is for everyone.

What is Best to Eat Before an Aerobic Workout?

Answer: Consider that you will probably burn between 300 and 450 kCal in an aerobic class. Keep the caloric content of the meal below that if you're intending to lose weight. That pretty much lets out any sort of "heavy" meal. The average American's diet is very high in protein, and relatively low in complex carbohydrates, so complex carbs before an aerobic workout are probably better. Keep the total calories from fat to 25% or lower, in general.

What is Best to Eat After an Aerobic Workout?

Answer: If you feel like eating immediately after a workout, be sure that it's high in carbohydrates, lower in protein, and has either very low or no fat content. The carbs should be mostly complex. Try to take in as few kCals as you can–just take the "edge" off. Munching out on broccoli or cauliflower salad with just a touch of fat-free margarine is good.

If the workout was pretty intense, I'd recommend about an hour's wait before eating a full meal. Most people aren't really ready to eat when they're sweaty and still breathing heavily, anyhow. Cool down, then grab a nice refreshing shower, and mellow out with a big glass of ice water. Next, find some candles, and sit down to a nice plate of rigatoni with tomato sauce with basil, green peppers, and a little bit of chopped mushrooms. Brush your whole wheat toast with a film of olive oil, sprinkle on some freshly-chopped garlic... you get the picture.

What is the Best Time of the Day to Exercise?

Answer: As a general rule, if your habits are diurnal, exercise in the early evening when your metabolism is at its peak, is more efficient. This varies widely, however, and you really need to exercise at the time which "feels" best for you. The best time to work out is when you want to, so pick a time of day at which you find exercise enjoyable.

Miscellaneous

What should I do to exercise safely?

In order to exercise safely, you should follow these tips:

1. Stop exercising right away if you:
    - Have pain or pressure in the left-chest or mid-chest area–or left neck, shoulder, or arm
    - Feel dizzy or sick
    - Break out in a cold sweat
    - Have muscle cramps
    - Feel pain in your joints, feet, ankles, or legs. You could hurt yourself if you ignore the pain.

(Ask your physician what to do if you have any of these symptoms.)

2. Slow down if out of breath. You should be able to talk while exercising without gasping for breath.
3. Drink lots of water before, during, and after exercise (even during workouts) to replace the water you lose by sweating.

4. Do not do hard exercise for 2 hours after a big meal (but a 5 to 10-minute walk is OK). If you eat small meals, you can exercise more often.
5. Wear the right clothes:
   - Wear lightweight, loose-fitting tops so you can move easily.
   - Wear supportive athletic shoes for weight-bearing activities.
   - Wear clothes made of fabrics that absorb sweat and remove it from your skin.
   - Never wear rubber or plastic suits. These could hold the sweat on your skin and make your body overheat.
   - Wear a knit hat to keep you warm when you exercise outdoors in cold weather.
   - Wear a cap in hot weather to help keep you cool.
   - Wear sunscreen when you exercise outdoors. Cover all areas of exposed skin.

OOO

Exercise Injuries, Reactions and Environment

Injuries and Syndromes

The following sections describe a number of injuries and syndromes that can befall the exerciser. While this information can be useful in determining appropriate first aid or symptomatic relief methods, it is important to be aware of the distinction between first aid and relief of symptoms vs. diagnosis and treatment.

As will become evident in the sections ahead, a single symptom (such as knee pain) can have a variety of causes, many of which are not immediately obvious and require the diagnosis of a physician, who can prescribe treatment.

Readers are strongly advised not to use the information below to "self-diagnose", but merely as guidelines for appropriate first aid/symptomatic relief and when to see a physician.

Legal Issues for the Exercise Professionals

Exercise professionals are strongly advised to refrain from the process of diagnosis and/or prescription of treatment or rehabilitative exercise. Remember, our scope of practice is limited to encouraging rest, RICE, and a visit to the doctor.

(RICE stands for Rest, Ice, Compression and Elevation.)

Statements such as, "That sounds like chondromalacia– why don't you try and strengthen the medical quad to help out” or “you’ve got low back syndrome” involve a judgment by the exercise professional that can be construed in a court of law as a diagnosis and/or prescription of rehabilitative exercise.

Exercise professionals are best advised to speak in general terms without reference to an individual’s condition, to focus on general preventive behaviour, and to refer individuals to a physician when a diagnosis needs to be made or an injury does not respond to first aid/symptomatic relief (such as RICE).

An appropriate example: “Well, there are a number of causes for the shin pain you’re experiencing. You can apply RICE to relieve the symptoms, but if it doesn’t feel better within a day or two you should consult with your physician.” Here, we sidestep the issue of diagnosis, stress symptomatic relief, and incorporate a physician referral in one sentence.

Or, “Now we’re going to do some exercises for the back. It is believed that strengthening the low back can help prevent low back pain.” In this case, only a general discussion on preventive (not rehabilitative) exercise is provided.

What should I do for an Acute Injury?

If you feel that you have “pulled a muscle” or have an inexplicable pain after exercising, the immediate treatment is RICE (rest, ice, compression, elevation). Icing for 48 hours, every 2 hours for about 10-15 minutes, should help the injured area. However, if you’ve got an injury that doesn’t respond to RICE in a couple of days, you should see your physician.

What should I do for a Chronic Injury?

You must see your physician or other qualified person to find out what you should do if an injury persists.

What are Common Exercise Injuries?

Overuse Injuries

The heading of overuse injuries is a broad one, into which the vast majority of exercise-related injuries fall. Generally, overuse injuries are chronic ones, meaning that no single event causes them (as with a sprained ankle or a broken leg), but a long series of events over weeks, months, or years of training gradually weaken or irritate the area in question until exercise becomes difficult or impossible, or other symptoms appear.

The vast majority of overuse injuries can be avoided by proper attention to form and technique, appropriate rest, proper equipment (especially footwear), and gradual increase of exercise frequency, intensity, and duration.

The best cures for an overuse injury are rest followed by a gradual return to activity, coupled with an awareness of the problem activity, and appropriate corrective measures (be they a more gradual return to exercise, appropriate strengthening, or avoidance of certain forms of activity).

Patellofemoral Syndrome ("Runner's Knee") / Chondromalacia

Chondromalacia literally refers to the wearing away of the cartilage on the back surface of the kneecap, which might be first exhibited as a "clicking" or "grating" sound, and knee pain under the patella (kneecap).

Chondromalacia refers to the condition, and not a specific disease state, as many possible causes exist for damage to the cartilage.

Patellofemoral syndrome, likewise, refers to generalized knee pain, often associated with runners, but not limited to runners alone. In this context, the cause is usually improper running mechanics over a period of time, though in many cases, the cause is unknown.

Once chondromalacia has occurred, the process is irreversible, and attention is paid to achieving the maximal amount of pain-free activity, and avoiding activities which will cause further damage to the joint.

Note that patellofemoral pain is of a more general nature, and may or may not be due to the pathological condition of chondromalacia.

It is best to consult a physician or a physical therapist when any sort of knee pain is encountered.

Plantar Fasciitis and Neuromas

Plantar fasciitis is literally an inflammation of the plantar fascia, a web of tough, fibrous connective tissue on the bottom of the foot. Neuromas are irritated nerve endings, but can cause pain in the foot (or other places, depending on the nerve in question).

Either condition should be examined by a physician. While both are commonly caused by overuse, the question of whether the condition is due to poor technique, simple overuse, or an orthopaedic problem, should be explored.

In the case of the latter, orthotics (inserts for shoes designed to help maintain proper impact cushioning and support for the foot) can play a major role in the prevention of future episodes.

Lateral Epicondylitis ("Tennis Elbow") and Tendonitis/Arthritis/Bursitis

Any "-itis" condition refers to inflammation or irritation. In the cases of tendonitis, arthritis, and bursitis, the sites of inflammation are the tendons, joints, and bursae (fluid-filled sacs provided cushioning between tendons and bones) respectively.

Again, any of these conditions should involve a physician referral. Tendonitis and bursitis are common overuse injuries, and rehabilitation will generally involve rest, and enhancing flexibility and strength of all muscles surrounding the joints near the area in question.

Arthritis can be caused by two distinct disease processes–osteoarthritis is essentially "wear and tear" on joints, in which the cartilage covering the articulating surfaces of the bones becomes worn and the joint reacts, often by swelling and filling with fluid. It can become quite tender, and motion can become difficult.

Rheumatoid arthritis is an auto-immune disorder in which the body launches an attack on its own joint tissues. While much less common than osteoarthritis, it can be severely debilitating.

Rehabilitation for arthritis generally involves activities that are low-impact in nature, and strengthening exercises. Activities are carried out through a "pain-free range of motion" (ROM limited by the onset of discomfort), and no activity is recommended during periods of active inflammation.

Shin Splints and Compartment Syndromes

Shin splints are a common name for pain felt in the anterior portion of the calf, which can be due to a variety of causes, from muscle imbalances to something as serious as a compartment syndrome.

Generally, treatment for shin splints involves RICE, strengthening exercises for all of the muscles surrounding the ankle joint, and flexibility exercises.

Compartment syndromes are a much less common, but more serious problem, where one of the compartments between muscles which contains blood vessels and/or nerves becomes swollen, compressing the blood vessels and/or nerves. This can lead to pain, swelling and discomfort, and in severe situations, can be an emergency situation requiring surgical intervention.

What are Some Common Exercise Reactions?

Some people experience reactions to exercise, ranging from uticaria, a harmless red blotchiness on the neck, face, or arms, to exercise-induced asthma or bronchospasm, to anaphylaxis.

Exercise-induced Asthma (EIA) is most likely to strike individuals exercising in cold, dusty, or excessively humid environments, and can range in severity from mild coughing to severe discomfort. Individuals who suspect that they have exercise-induced Asthma, are encouraged to seek medical attention to rule out other possibilities, and to ensure the best possible treatment for their condition.

General recommendations for persons with EIA include an extended warm-up, avoidance of cold, dusty, or extremely humid environments for exercise, pursed-lip breathing, and keeping an inhaler handy for use during exercise (if recommended by physician).

While very rare, it is possible for someone to have an allergic reaction to exercise, called Exercise-Induced Anaphylaxis (EIA). This is a life-threatening situation, and requires immediate medical attention. People prone to EIA can, at the advice of their physicians, carry a bee-sting kit to use in such situations. Any person suspecting being prone to EIA, should consult their physician before resuming exercise.

Some Common Environmental Concerns

Extremes of temperature and humidity pose special problems for the exerciser. In hot weather, care must be taken to wear clothing that is light, breathes well, and allows for the evaporation of sweat.

"Sauna suits", "tummy wraps", and other products designed to encourage quick weight loss through sweat are particularly dangerous–the body can reach dangerous (or even fatal) core temperatures in very short periods of time. Weight lost by these methods will be regained as soon as water is ingested again, and so the risk outweighs any benefit.

On extremely humid days, care must be taken to exercise at an appropriately lowered intensity, out of the high heat/ humidity, or even to postpone exercise until the heat/ humidity diminishes. As exercise intensity increases and more heat must be dissipated, evaporation of sweat becomes the principal means by which cooling occurs. In a high-humidity environment, evaporation becomes less effective at cooling, and the risk of heat-related injury is greater.

Adequate hydration is also the key to safe exercise in the heat, as the body will produce large quantities of sweat. One or two cups of water before exercise and a cup of water during exercise are recommended, though more can be ingested.

It is important to remember that the thirst mechanism lags behind the body's need for fluid – by the time one is thirsty one is already substantially dehydrated. Even small amounts of dehydration can affect performance and severe dehydration can be life-threatening.

Contrary to popular belief, water consumed during exercise will not contribute to cramping, so "swish and spit" should be avoided in favour of consuming small amounts of water steadily during the exercise session, especially during periods of prolonged exercise.

In the cold, care must be taken as well. It is best to dress in layers that will wick sweat away from the body–many of the "high-tech" fabrics that are now available, will do this admirably. Outer layers can be used to keep the body warm during a warm-up and removed as exercise progresses to allow the body to cool itself, and then be replaced during the cooldown to avoid an excessive chill.

Garments made of fabrics like wool, which will insulate even when wet, are superior to garments made of materials like cotton, which will contain sweat and can contribute to heat lost by evaporation and conduction as the activity level decreases.

Heat-Related Problems and Injuries

Who is at Risk for Heat-Related Illness?

People at risk for heat-related illnesses include those who work or exercise outdoors, elderly people, young children, and people with health problems. Also at risk are those who have had a heat-related illness in the past, those with medical conditions that cause poor blood circulation, and those who take medications to get rid of water (diuretics).

People usually try to get out of extreme heat before they begin to feel ill. However, some people do not or cannot. Athletes and those who work outdoors often keep working even after they begin to feel ill. Those living in poorly ventilated or poorly insulated or poorly heated buildings are at risk of heat emergencies. Many times, they might not even recognize that they are in danger of becoming ill.

What are Heat-Related Illnesses?

Heat cramps, heat exhaustion, and heat stroke are conditions caused by over-exposure to heat.

HEAT CRAMPS are the least severe, and often are the first signals that the body is having trouble with the heat. Heat cramps are painful muscle spasms. They usually occur in the legs and abdomen. Think of them as a warning of a possible heat-related emergency.

HEAT EXHAUSTION is a more severe condition than heat cramps. It often affects athletes, fire fighters, construction workers, and factory workers, as well as those who wear heavy clothing in hot, humid environments. Its signals include cool, moist, pale or flushed skin, headache, nausea, dizziness, weakness, and exhaustion.

HEAT STROKE is the least common but most severe heat emergency. It most often occurs when people ignore the signals of heat exhaustion. Heat stroke develops when the body systems are overwhelmed by heat and begin to stop functioning. Heat stroke is a serious medical emergency. The signals of heat stroke include red, hot, dry skin; changes in consciousness; rapid, weak pulse; and rapid, shallow breathing.

How to Treat Heat Cramps?

To care for HEAT CRAMPS, have the victim rest in a cool place. Give him cool water or a commercial sports drink. Usually, rest and fluids are all the person needs to recover.

Lightly stretch and gently massage the area. The victim should not take salt tablets or salt water. This can make the situation worse.

When the cramps stop, the person can usually start activity again if there are no other signals of illness. He should keep drinking plenty of fluids. Watch the victim carefully for further signals of heat-related illness.

How to Treat Other Heat-Related Illnesses?

When you recognize heat-related illness in its early stages, you can usually reverse it. Get the victim out of the heat. Loosen any tight clothing and apply cool, wet clothes. If the victim is conscious, give him cool water to drink.

DO NOT let the conscious victim drink too quickly. Give about one glass (4 ounces) of water every 15 minutes. Let the victim rest in a comfortable position and watch carefully for changes in his condition. The victim should not resume normal activities the same day.

At What Temperatures and Humidity are Heat-Related Illnesses Likely?

According to 1993 American Red Cross Standard First Aid Manual:

- ***Hot:*** {93°F (34°C), 20% humidity}, {87°F (31°C), 50%}, {82°F (28°C), 100%} Sunstroke, heat cramps, or heat exhaustion possible with prolonged exposure/exercise
- ***Very Hot:*** {105°F (41°C), 20%}, {92°F (34°C), 60%}, {87°F (31°C), 100%} Heat cramps or heat exhaustion likely
- ***Extremely Hot:*** {120°F (49°C), 20%}, {108°F (43°C), 40%}, {91°F (33°C), 100%} Heat Stroke or sun stroke imminent

Reference, 1993 American Red Cross Standard First Aid Manual

Specific Cold-Related Injuries—Hypothermia and Frostbite

Frostbite involves the freezing of tissue, and can range from mild to fairly severe. The skin generally looks yellowish, and will be cold to the touch. First aid generally involves warming the affected area using moderately warm water–remember that sensation will be reduced in the area, and the temperature of the water should be verified by running it on unaffected skin! DO NOT rub the area, as this can cause further tissue damage.

Frostbite should be examined by a physician to assess the extent of the damage. It is best prevented by proper clothing and limited exposure to cold.

Hypothermia is a life-threatening condition wherein the core body temperature has become dangerously low. Many of the same symptoms as heat exhaustion, including dizziness, nausea, loss of appetite, vision problems, etc., may be present. In the case of hypothermia, it is important to use any means available to warm the victim, such as removing excess clothing and putting them in a sleeping bag with an unaffected person who can provide body warmth until other medical aids arrive.

OOO

Daily Caloric Requirements

A pound is equivalent to 3500 calories. To over simplify, if you want to lose one pound per week, reduce your caloric consumption by 3500 calories per week. Consuming less than 1500 calories per day on a regular basis reduces the basal metabolic rate. When the metabolic rate is reduced, fewer calories can be consumed. Excess calories will be stored as fat. This is why it's important to combine exercise with diet in order to affect weight loss.

Your basal metabolic rate is the basic minimum number of calories that are required to maintain your body weight based on average body composition. To calculate your basal metabolic rate:

Basal Metabolic Rate (BMR) = 24 * Weight (lb)/2.2

OR

Basal Metabolic Rate (BMR) = 24 * Weight (kg)

The BMR is then multiplied by a number representing the individuals activity level:

Sedentary	Light	Medium	Heavy
BMR * 1.45	BMR * 1.60	BMR * 1.70	BMR * 1.88

Generally, eating more than this number of calories increases weight and less than this number allows weight reduction. However, BMR does not take into account extremes of activity or inactivity. Therefore, BMR should be used as an approximation. Various activities will increase caloric requirements above the BMR. The following table shows the approximate amount of calories required for a 135-pound individual performing the following listed activity for 1 hour:

Activity	Calories Expended	Activity	Calories Expended
Aerobics	620	Bicycling 12mph	620
Running 5mph	500	Ski Machine	550
Walking 4mph	230	Swimming	470
Soccer	370	Stair Master	350

Dietary Requirements of Protein, Carbohydrate and Fat

Proper nutrition requires a balanced intake of Proteins, Carbohydrates and Fats. Proteins and Carbohydrates are both 4 calories per gram. Fat is 9 calories per gram. An example follows for a daily caloric requirement of 2000 calories. The amount of grams of each will vary according to your daily caloric requirement (based on BMR). However, the percentage should remain the same for all. The following example is for a daily calorie requirement of 2000 calories:

- Protein 4 cal/g 30% of total = 600 cal (protein) = 150g
- Carbohydrates 4 cal/g 60% of total = 1200 cal (carbs) = 300g
- Fat 9 cal/g 10% of total = 200 cal (fat) = 22g

Fats, Oils & Sweets
USE SPARINGLY

Milk, Yogurt & Cheese Group
2-3 SERVINGS

Meal, Poultry, Fish, Dry Beans Eggs & Nuts Group
2-3 SERVINGS

Vegetable Group
3-5 SERVINGS

Fruit Group
2-3 SERVINGS

Bread, Cereal, Rice & Pasta Group
6-11 SERVINGS

Food Pyramid Guide

USDA RDA/DRI

Female Age	9 - 14	15 – 18	19 - 24	25 - 50	51+
Calories	2200 kcal	2200 kcal	2200 kcal	2200 kcal	1900 kcal
Protein	46 g	44 g	46 g	50 g	50 g
Calcium	1300 mg	1300 mg	1000 mg	1000 mg	1200 mg
Iron	15 mg	15 mg	15 mg	15 mg	10 mg
Sodium	500 mg	500 mg	500 mg	500 mg	500 mg
Phosphorus	1250 mg	1250 mg	700 mg	700 mg	700 mg
Vitamin A	2600 IU	2600 IU	2600 IU	2600 IU	2600 IU
Vitamin C	50 mg	60 mg	60 mg	60 mg	60 mg
Vitamin D	5 ug	5 ug	5 ug	5 ug	10 ug
Thiamin	1.1 mg	1.1 mg	1.1 mg	1.1 mg	1.0 mg
Riboflavin	1.3 mg	1.3 mg	1.3 mg	1.3 mg	1.2 mg
Niacin	15 mg	15 mg	15 mg	15 mg	13 mg

Male Age	11 - 14	15 - 18	19 - 24	25 - 50	51+
Calories	2500 kcal	3000 kcal	2900 kcal	2900 kcal	2300 kcal
Protein	45 g	59 g	58 g	63 g	63 g
Calcium	1300 mg	1300 mg	1000 mg	1000 mg	1200 mg
Iron	12 mg	12 mg	10 mg	10 mg	10 mg
Sodium	500 mg	500 mg	500 mg	500 mg	500 mg
Phosphorus	1250 mg	1250 mg	700 mg	700 mg	700 mg
Vitamin A	3300 IU	3300 IU	3300 IU	3300 IU	3300 IU
Vitamin C	50 mg	60 mg	60 mg	60 mg	60 mg
Vitamin D	5 ug	5 ug	5 ug	5 ug	5 ug
Thiamin	1.3 mg	1.5 mg	1.5 mg	1.5 mg	1.2 mg
Riboflavin	1.5 mg	1.8 mg	1.7 mg	1.7 mg	1.4 mg
Niacin	17 mg	20 mg	19 mg	19 mg	15 mg

Child Age	0 - 0.5	0.5 - 1	1 - 3	4 - 6	7 - 10
Calories	650 kcal	850 kcal	1300 kcal	1800 kcal	2000 kcal
Protein	13 g	14 g	16 g	24 g	28 g
Calcium	210 mg	270 mg	500 mg	800 mg	1000 mg
Iron	6 mg	10 mg	10 mg	10 mg	10 mg
Sodium	120 mg	200 mg	300 mg	400 mg	400 mg
Phosphorus	300 mg	500 mg	800 mg	800 mg	800 mg
Vitamin A	1200 IU	1200 IU	1300 IU	1600 IU	2300 IU
Vitamin C	30 mg	35 mg	40 mg	45 mg	45 mg
Vitamin D	5 ug	5 ug	5 ug	5 ug	5 ug
Thiamin	0.3 mg	0.4 mg	0.7 mg	0.9 mg	1 mg
Riboflavin	0.4 mg	0.5 mg	0.8 mg	1.1 mg	1.2 mg
Niacin	5 mg	6 mg	9 mg	12 mg	13 mg

1 microgram (ug) = 3.3 IU

Source: US Department of Agriculture

OOO

Glossary

ATP: A complicated chemical formed with energy released from food. Stored in muscle cells. From the breakdown of ATP, energy is released for a cell to perform work.

Aerobic: In the presence of oxygen.

Anaerobic: In the absence of oxygen.

Artery: A vessel carrying blood away from the heart.

ATP-PC System: Anaerobic energy system where ATP is manufactured when PC (Phosphocretine) is broken down. Activity performed at maximum output for less than 15 seconds derives energy from the ATP-PC System.

Bioenergetics: The study of energy transformations.

Blood Pressure: The force moving blood through the circulatory system.

Calorie: A non-metric measurement unit of energy. One calorie is the energy required to raise the temperature of one gram of water by 1 degree Celsius.
1 calorie = 4.2 kilojoules.

Capillary: A small blood vessel situated in the network between veins and arteries, where exchange of gases, food fuel, waste products etc. between blood and tissue takes place.

Carbohydrate: One of the groups of chemical compounds, which contain carbon, hydrogen and oxygen. Found in food.

Cardiac Cycle: contraction (Systole) and relaxation (Diastole) of the heart.

Cardiac Output: The amount of blood pumped by the heart in 1 minute.

Central Nervous System: Brain and spinal column nervous tissue.

Conduction: Transfer of heat between two objects in contact.

Diastole: The resting part of the cardiac cycle.

Eccentric Contraction: When the muscle gets longer while still contracting.

Energy: The capacity to perform work.

Ergometer: A type of exercise bike or similar exercise machine used for measuring physiological effects of exercise on the human body.

Evaporation: Loss of heat resulting from change of fluid into a vapour.

Fat: (1) *(Food)* Glycerol plus fatty acids, a basic foodstuff.

(2) *(On the body)* Greasy white and yellow substance under the skin *(and elsewhere)* where food is stored for future energy needs.

Fitness: The ability of the body to cope with stress.

Flexibility: The range of motion through a joint.

Fulcrum: The point of rotation in the lever system.

Glucose: A sugar.

Glycogen: The form sugar takes when stored in the body as e.g. liver glycogen or muscle glycogen.

Golgi Tendon Organ: A kinematic sense organ situated in the juncture between muscle and tendon.

Heat: A form of energy.

Heat Exhaustion: Fatigue caused by being in a hot environment.

Heat Stroke: Potentially fatal illness which results from over-exposure to excessive heat conditions.

Humidity: Moisture held in the air.

Hypertension: High blood pressure.

Hypertrophy: Increase in size of an organ e.g. muscular hypertrophy in muscles.

Hypotension: Low blood pressure.

Isokinetic Contraction: Muscular contraction where tension is maintained maximally over the complete range of motion.

Isometric Contraction: Muscular contraction where tension is maintained but the muscle stays at the same length.

Isotonic Contraction: Muscular contraction where a muscle contracts and shortens–variable tension but a constant load.

Joint Receptors: Sense organs concerned with telling you where your 'body' is in relation to your environment (kinesthesis).

Kilojoules: Metric measurement unit of energy. 1 Kilojoule (kJ) = 0.24 calories.

Kreb's Cycle: An aerobic energy system in your body which uses oxygen and food to produce ATP.

Lactic Acid System: An anaerobic energy system in which ATP is produced from the breakdown of sugar into lactic acid. Requires no oxygen.

Metabolism: Chemical changes in your body which use food fuels and oxygen to liberate energy for work, heat etc.

Mitochondria: A cell 'organelle' in which KREB'S CYCLE takes place. Their number can increase with physical training, and they are found in aerobic cells like muscle cells.

Muscle Spindle: Sense organs inside muscles.

Oxygen System: Aerobic energy system which produces abundant ATP in comparison to other energy systems. Food (sugar and fat) is broken down and, in the presence of oxygen, ATP can be manufactured. This energy is used during endurance activities, which take in excess of 10 minutes to complete (e.g. long distance running.)

Phosphocreation (PC): Chemical compound kept in muscle cells which helps in the manufacture of ATP.

Protein: One of the basic foods we eat.

Receptor: A sense organ e.g. the heat receptor, can 'sense' heat.

Respiratory Exchange Ratio: The ratio of carbon dioxide produced to the oxygen consumed:

Carbon Dioxide Produced per minute
Oxygen Consumed per minute

Strength: The force that a muscle can exert in one big effort.

Stroke Volume: The amount of blood pumped by the heart per beat.

Temperature: The degree of heat or cold.

Vasoconstriction: Decrease in the diameter of a blood vessel, thereby causing reduced blood flow to the area supplied by that blood vessel (normally an artery).

Work: Application of force through a distance.

OOO